A Layn

Chronic
Diseases

A Layman's Guide to
Chronic
Diseases

M.K. Gupta

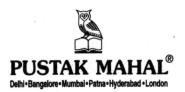

PUSTAK MAHAL®
Delhi•Bangalore•Mumbai•Patna•Hyderabad•London

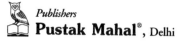

Publishers

Pustak Mahal®, Delhi

J-3/16 , Daryaganj, New Delhi-110002
☎ 23276539, 23272783, 23272784 • *Fax:* 011-23260518
E-mail: info@pustakmahal.com • *Website:* www.pustakmahal.com

London Office
5, Roddell Court, Bath Road, Slough SL3 OQJ, England
E-mail: pustakmahaluk@pustakmahal.com

Sales Centre
10-B, Netaji Subhash Marg, Daryaganj, New Delhi-110002
☎ 23268292, 23268293, 23279900 • *Fax:* 011-23280567
E-mail: rapidexdelhi@indiatimes.com

Branch Offices
Bangalore: ☎ 22234025
E-mail: pmblr@sancharnet.in • pustak@sancharnet.in
Mumbai: ☎ 22010941
E-mail: rapidex@bom5.vsnl.net.in
Patna: ☎ 3294193 • *Telefax:* 0612-2302719
E-mail: rapidexptn@rediffmail.com
Hyderabad: *Telefax:* 040-24737290
E-mail: pustakmahalhyd@yahoo.co.in

© **Author**

ISBN 978-81-223-0128-1

5th Edition : February 2007

Printed at : Unique Colour Carton, Mayapuri, Delhi-110064

Preface

Chronic diseases are continually on the increase in our society. Medical science has no permanent answer for it. It can only provide symptomatic and temporary relief which, though, itself is a good thing but not an ultimate answer to these problems.

This is where Yoga and Naturecure come to the rescue. It is a matter of pleasure that awareness of the people in this direction is gradually increasing, though, still it is much less than what it should be.

The present book is a humble attempt in this direction. However, the special feature of the book is that it first explains the nature of disease in detail in a scientific manner and then discusses about the causes, prevention and cure mainly based on Yoga and Naturecure. It constantly maintains a scientific approach so that the reader can fully appreciate as to what and why he is doing. However, I must mention that this book is a general layman's guide and not a substitute for the advice of a Medical or a Naturecure expert and one must consult them when so warranted.

I would like to apologize for any mistakes in the book and will appreciate reader's comments and suggestions.

With best wishes for the readers.

—M.K. Gupta
Inter-University Accelerator Centre
(Formerly Nuclear Science Centre)
J.N.U. Campus, New Delhi-110067
Tel: 26892601, 26892603
E-mail: *mkg@iuac.ernet.in*

Contents

1. High Blood Pressure

What Does Blood Pressure Mean?

Blood pressure (B.P.) is merely the pressure that the blood exerts on the blood vessels while circulating. An optimum amount of B.P. is essential for:

a. the return of the blood to the heart, after making its way through more than 60,000 miles long blood vessels of our body

b. the exchange of nutrients and waste products between the various cells of the body and the blood capillaries

c. the filtering and therefore purification of the blood in kidneys and lungs.

At every contraction, the heart pumps about 70 ml of blood into the arteries. This quantity is termed as 'stroke volume'. Thus it pumps about 5 litres of blood every minutes. (It is also the total quantity of blood in an adult's body). This quantity is termed as cardiac output (or CMO).

Cardiac output (CMO) = stroke volume x heart rate

Every time your heart beats, it pumps out blood. This blood flows through three types of blood vessels: the arteries, the capillaries and the veins in this order and returns to the heart again. When the doctor talks to you about B.P., he usually means the pressure of the flowing blood in the arteries. Usually the pressure the heart exerts to send blood throughout the body is 120 mm Hg. However, the pressure of the blood returning to the heart is nearly zero. The difference in this pressure causes blood to circulate through the body. The pressure gradually decreases while circulating.

Systolic and Diastolic B.P.

When the rhythmically beating heart contracts, it forcefully drives the blood into the arteries. The pressure at such a time is high and is termed 'Systolic Blood Pressure'. At this time the elastic walls of the large arteries expand.

When the heart relaxes to be filled with blood from various parts of the body, the pressure is minimum in the arteries and is termed 'Diastolic B.P.' At this time, the elastic walls of the large arteries recoil. This recoil continues to push the blood forward against the resistance offered by the arterioles.

How B.P. is Measured

B.P. is usually measured in the **'Brachial'** artery of your arm using an instrument known as **'Sphygmomanometer'**. This is because there is no difference in the blood pressure between your upper arm and at the 'aorta' where the blood leaves the heart. For many decades, B.P. has been recorded in mm on a mercury column (mm Hg). In recent times, sphygmomano meters without mercury columns (aneroid and digital instruments) are also used. They too express the readings as mm of Hg.

Mercury sphygmomanometer consists of a rubber bag encased in a fabric(cloth) cuff. A rubber tube connects the bag with the mercury column. A second rubber tube leads to bulb by which the bag is inflated to constrict the arm artery. When the artery is compressed, the blood flow there stops. Gradual release of the air in the cuff results in partial opening of the artery causing a turbulent flow of blood. The point at which the blood begins to flow is heard by the doctor as distinct thumping sound through a stethoscope placed over the artery. The reading on the sphygmomanometer at this point indicates your systolic pressure. Further gradual release of air from the cuff reduces pressure on the artery till it opens completely and the blood flows normally. The sounds of turbulent blood flow therefore disappear. The reading on sphygmomanometer at this point denotes your diastolic B.P.

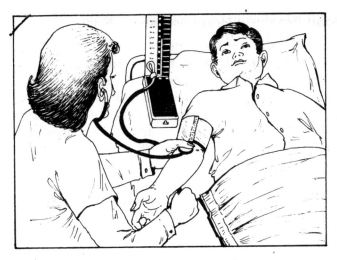

Fig. 1.1

Precautions while Taking B.P. Measurement

1. Measure your B.P. when you are relaxed, 1–2 hours after eating, several minutes after urination, with the room temperature of about 20°C.

2. Don't proceed with the measurement until your breathing pattern is back to normal. B.P. is stabilized by deeply breathing 5–6 times before measurement.

3. Don't measure continuously over a long period of time. Even when taking 2–3 readings simultaneously, wait for a while before taking another B.P. measurement. Waiting allows the engorged blood vessels to return to normal. Two readings three minutes apart are desirable especially for those under stress.

4. Don't increase abdominal pressure. The B.P. may become higher if you bend the back (e.g. when sitting on a chair and using a low table for measurement) B.P. may also become higher if you cross your legs while sitting on a chair or you are sitting cross legged on the floor.

5. If you measure B.P. while lying down, the measured B.P. may differ from the one measured while sitting.

6. The cuff should be at the level of heart.

Blood Pressure Homeostasis in Body

The vasomotor centre of the brain corrects the sudden changes in your B.P. without your knowledge. This is done by adjusting the peripheral resistance (resistance to the blood flow due to friction between blood and walls of blood vessels) and/or cardiac output. Change in either of these two factors modifies the B.P. because B.P. is directly proportional to cardiac output and peripheral resistance. When B.P. rises, the vasomotor centre sends messages to the arterioles (small branches of arteries) to relax. The peripheral resistance decreases and B.P. reaches normal level. Similarly when the B.P. falls, the vasomotor centre sends messages to the arterioles to contract. Thus the peripheral resistance increases. The vasomotor centre also increases the cardiac output by increasing the activity of the heart. The combination of increased peripheral resistance and cardiac output increases the B.P. and it reaches normal levels.

What are Normal Blood Pressure Values?

The normal adult systolic pressure ranges from 120-140 mm of Hg. The normal adult diastolic pressure ranges from 80-90 mm of Hg depending upon age (Refer Table 1.1 at the end of this chapter).

As a thumb rule you can calculate your average ideal B.P. by the following formula:

Systolic B.P.   For age 20-60 yrs. = 120 + 1/5th of age
For age above 60 = 135 + 1 for each year above 60

Diastolic B.P.   At age 25 yrs. = 80
For age above 25 yrs. = 80 + 1 for every 5 years beyond the age of 25 yrs.

Blood Pressure Variations

Blood pressure values don't remain same throughout the day. B.P. is usually lower in the early mornings and higher in the late evenings. It is least when the person is in deep sleep or deep relaxation. Physical exercise, emotional stress or physical pain increase the blood pressure temporarily. B.P. tends to be higher in cold weather and lower in warm weather. At higher altitudes also, B.P. tends to rise.

Temporary Conditions which Lead to Increase in B.P.

Blood pressure becomes higher if you are

- Mentally stressed, anxious, impatient
- Constipated
- In cold weather

B.P. becomes temporarily higher after

- Eating
- Drinking coffee, tea, alcohol
- Bathing or showering
- Exercises
- Smoking
- Urination

What is High Blood Pressure (or Hypertension)

Hypertension in adults means (a) persistent systolic pressure of 140 mm of Hg or more or (b) a persistent diastolic pressure of 90 mm of Hg or more. Until recently systolic pressure more than 160 mm of Hg was defined as hypertension. However the World Health Organization has now recommended that a persistent systolic pressure between 140 and 160 mm of Hg should also be considered as hypertension. (For classification of mild, moderate and severe hypertension, refer Table 1.2 at the end of this chapter).

Levels of Diastolic B.P. is considered more important in the diagnosis of H.B.P. because this shows the minimum pressure sustained by the artery walls continuously.

When a person has got High B.P., it only means that now heart has to exert greater force to pump almost the same quantity of blood within the same time due to which B.P. becomes elevated than normal.

Causes of Hypertension

1. Heredity
2. Mental tension
3. Excess intake of salt
4. Obesity
5. Sedentary life
6. Smoking
7. Alcohol
8. Diet having saturated fats (see Table 1.4 of the book)
9. Use of fried and too much oily foods
10. Excess intake of sugar
11. Diabetes
12. Tea, coffee, cold drinks (having caffeine).

Many of the above factors lead to narrowing and hardening of the arteries (atherosclerosis) because of deposition of cholesterol in the walls of the arteries. As old age approaches, the artery walls harden and lose much of their elasticity. This is the reason why elderly people have a higher blood pressure than young people. When arteries become narrow and hard (i.e. loss of elasticity to expand and contract), the blood has to be pushed through greater force by heart leading to High B.P.

Blood lipids (cholesterol and triglycerides) are required to be kept within desirable limits to avoid their deposition in the arteries (Refer Table 1.3 at the end of this chapter in this regard).

Some Quantitative Facts about Developing Primary Hypertension

1. A person with sedentary life style is twenty to fifty percent greater risk of developing hypertension
2. An overweight person is at two to six times the higher risk of developing hypertension. A higher waist to hip ratio is more frequently associated with hypertension
3. If one parent has hypertension, the children are at thirty percent greater risk of developing hypertension
4. If both the parents have hypertension, the children are at forty percent greater risk of developing hypertension

5. People who are sensitive to salt intake are at risk of developing hypertension if they take more than 5–6 grams of salt per day.

Types of Hypertension

High Blood Pressure is of two types

1. Essential (or primary) hypertension
2. Secondary hypertension.

The matter in this chapter deals mainly with essential hypertension. Secondary hypertension is caused by some disease or disorder in the body e.g.

a. Diseases of the kidneys and endocrine glands– especially the adrenal glands
b. Long standing diabetes mellitus
c. Long term use of oral contraceptives containing oestrogen
d. Use of steroids for many years (steroids are a group of drugs commonly used for treatment of asthma, some skin disorders etc.)
e. Inborn defects of the 'aorta'
f. Pregnancy related disorders, especially during the last three months of pregnancy or immediately after delivery.

Risks Associated with Hypertension

1. **Angina Pectoris & Heart Attack:** It is characterized by severe pain in the chest region because coronary arteries supplying blood to the heart become narrow and don't expand during physical activity (because of atherosclerosis leading to narrowing and hardening of arteries), while the heart, at the same time, requires more blood. If the process of atherosclerosis goes unabated, a coronary artery may become too narrow and may get totally blocked. This results in heart attack.

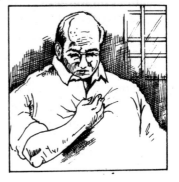

Fig. 1.2

The blood vessels of a healthy person are highly elastic and expand and contract accordingly as per the need of the blood requirement for an organ but in the case of High B.P. patient, they become narrow as well as hardened. *It is to be noted that atherosclerosis not only causes High B.P. but it is other way round also i.e High B.P. (caused due to any other reason) will also aggravate process of atherosclerosis. The proof to this claim is the fact that pulmonary arteries where the B.P. is as low as 35/15, never develop atherosclerosis.*

2. **Stroke (Brain Haemorrhage):** Atherosclerosis also renders the blood vessels brittle. If a brittle brain artery ruptures due to High pressure in the artery, it is termed as 'Stroke' (bleeding in the brain). It may also lead to paralysis of some portion of the body.

3. **Heart Failure:** When B.P. is high, the heart has to work harder. To perform the increased work, the heart muscle thickens and increases in size. The enlargement of the heart is visible in X-rays. For a period of time, despite the increased work load, the heart does well. But there comes a time when it tires and is not able to meet the strain. The result is congestive heart failure. In this situation, the heart doesn't stop beating but its contractions are weak. With each contraction less volume of blood is supplied, so less blood reaches the tissues of the body and the whole body starts suffering. For example reduced blood supply to legs may lead to early pain and fatigue in legs on walking.

4. **Effect on Kidneys:** If the B.P. rises, kidneys can't perform their work of blood filtration effectively. Consequently salts and toxins accumulate in the body. Each gm of salt accumulated in the body has a capacity to hold back 70 gm of water from being excreted. Such water retention aggravates heart failure. High B.P. also gradually destroys the cells of kidneys. Kidney damage is identified by loss of useful nutrients through the urine.

5. Eyes are also one of the target organs under attack in H.B.P.

Laboratory Tests for Ascertaining the Harms Done by Hypertension

1. Blood tests to identify diabetes, high cholesterol levels and defects in kidney function
2. Urine tests to detect diabetes and damage to the kidneys
3. ECG to detect changes in the heart
4. Chest X-ray to identify enlargement of the heart or the aorta.

Common Symptoms of Hypertensive Patients

1. Lack of sleep
2. headaches, especially throbbing pain, which is associated with anger and working under stress
3. dizziness
4. Flushed face on exertion
5. Excessive craving for salt
6. Obesity
7. Increased irritability and tendency to become angry or violent
8. Hurry and impatience and always racing against time.

A rapid or sudden increase in B.P. to very high levels (usually 240/140 mm of Hg or more) frequently leads to severe headaches, blurring of vision, drowsiness, vomitting and breathlessness. This requires emergency treatment.

Control of Hypertension

1. **Weight Reduction:** Your B.P. will fall by about 1.5 mm of Hg for every kg of weight loss.
2. **Reduction of Salt Intake:** (not more than 5–6 gm of salt per day). B.P. patients can use potassium salt instead sodium salt. To reduce salt intake, limit eating processed, canned foods, pickles, chutneys, papads, salted peanuts, wafers, potato chips etc. as they contain lot of salt.
3. **Aerobic Exercises:** Walking, running, swimming, cycling, sports etc. can reduce your resting blood pressure by 5–10 mm of Hg. This happens because of two reasons. First by aerobic exercises, arteries are dilated, so heart has

to apply less pressure to send the same amount of blood. Secondly, aerobic exercises increase HDL cholesterol (good cholesterol) and reduce harmful (LDL) cholesterol in blood which leads to reduction in blood pressure applied by the heart.

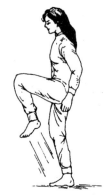

4. **Yogasanas and Stretching Exercises:** They relax muscles and promote free flow of blood leading to lowering of B.P. However, those exercises in which body is held upside down or the head remains below the level of heart for some time and those exercises which require holding of breath for some time, should be avoided.

Fig. 1.3 Aerobic exercises strengthen heart and reduce B.P.

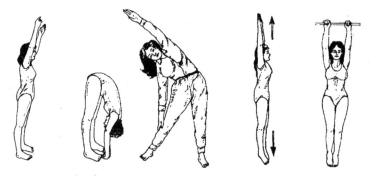

Fig. 1.4 Stretching exercises are good for a High B.P. patient

Note: Avoid isometric exercises like weight-lifting because they increase B.P. and do more harm than good.

5. Reduce Alcohol intake
6. Stop smoking
7. Reduce intake of sugar, coffee, tea, cola drinks
8. **Avoid Saturated Fats:** Limit food having saturated fats (egg, meat, ghee, butter, whole milk, cream, biscuits, cake, ice-creams, pastries, chocolates etc.) as these increase blood cholesterol. For list of foods having saturated and unsaturated foods and cholesterol content of various saturated foods, please refer to Tables 1.4 to 1.7.

9. **Calcium, Potassium and Magnesium:** They have been found to reduce B.P. Hence foods rich in these minerals should be taken. For example, lemon, banana, potato, peas, broccoli, tomato, cauliflower, sprouts and orange are good sources of potassium.

10. **High Intake of Fibres (Soluble Fibres):** Apple, banana, orange, potato, carrot, tomato, cabbage, beans are good sources of such fibres. Soluble fibre binds to dietary cholesterol and gets it excreted out of body and so indirectly helps in reducing B.P.

11. **Vitamins:** Vitamin C, vitamin B3 (Niacin) and vitamin E are considered good for lowering B.P.

12. **Special Food Items:** Some special food items like garlic, amla, honey, lemon juice, onion are considered very effective in lowering High B.P.

13. **Relaxation Techniques:** Any technique which reduces mental stress and promotes physical and mental relaxation (e.g. massage, music, meditation, humour/laughter, savasana, lying or walking in fresh air in a garden etc.) helps in reduction of High B.P.

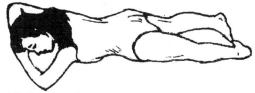

Fig. 1.5 Savasana (in prone position) for inducing relaxation

14. **Intake of Water:** Drink lot of water and more so in the morning in empty stomach. This helps to keep the blood thinner and reduces blood clotting tendency.

15. **General Change in Outlook towards Life:** If one makes his outlook towards life a positive one, then he won't be stressed by life's incidents so easily and therefore his B.P. will not rise because of mental stress.

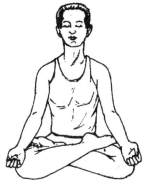

Fig. 1.6 Meditation is very helpful for High B.P. patient

19

16. 'Vayan' Mudra: There is one 'Mudra' in Yoga called 'Vayan Mudra' which is said to be effective for reducing high blood pressure if practiced off and on. In this mudra tips of forefinger and middle finger are joined to the tip of thumb.

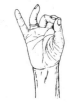

Fig. 1.7 Vayan Mudra

USEFUL TABLES

Table 1.1 Desirable Blood Pressure Values

Age	Systolic Range			Diastolic Range			Pulse-
(Years)	Min.	Avr.	Max.	Min.	Avr.	Max.	Pressure
15–19	105	117	120	73	77	81	40
20–24	108	120	132	75	79	83	41
25–29	109	121	133	76	80	84	41
30–34	110	122	134	77	81	85	41
35–39	110	123	135	78	82	86	41
40–44	112	125	137	79	83	87	42
45–49	115	127	139	80	84	88	43
50–54	116	129	142	81	85	89	44
55–59	118	131	144	82	86	90	45
60–64	121	134	147	83	87	91	47

Average Desirable Blood Pressure

For young people : 120/80

For old people : 140/90

Note: Pulse pressure is difference of systolic B.P. (Avr.) – Diastolic B.P. (Avr.)

Table 1.2 Unsafe Levels of Blood Pressure

Level of Severity	Systolic B.P.	Diastolic B.P.
Mild Hypertension	140–160	90–100
Moderate Hypertension	160–200	100–120
Severe Hypertension	Above 200	Above 120

Table 1.3 Blood Lipids Chart (mg/100 ml plasma)

Type of lipids	Desirable	Borderline High	High Risk
Total Cholesterol	<200	200–240	>240
LDL Cholesterol	<130	130–160	>160
HDL Cholesterol	>50	50–35	<35
Triglycerides	<150	150–500	>500

Table 1.4 Foods Containing Saturated and Unsaturated Fats

Fatty foods containing mainly saturated fats	Fatty foods containing mainly unsaturated fats
a) Butter, ghee (clarified butter), vegetable ghee (Vanaspati ghee or Dalda), coconut oil, palm oil	a) Vegetable oils: Peanut oil, sesame oil, maize oil, soya bean oil, karadi oil, cottonseed oil, sunflower oil and dishes prepared from these oils
b) Whole milk, cream, khoya, khoya-based preparations, sweets prepared in ghee and vegetable ghee, whole-milk preparations (shreekhand, basudi, ice cream, pedas, etc.), cheese	b) Nuts: Almonds, Cashew-nuts, Peanuts, Walnuts, Pistachio etc.
c) Chocolates, cakes, biscuits, wafers	c) All Cereals and Pulses
d) Egg, meat, oysters, fish	

Table 1.5 Fat Contents of Commonly Used Vegetable Oils & Ghee (in%)

Type of Oils/Ghee	Saturated Fat	Monoun-saturated Fat (Oleic Acid)	Polyunsaturated Fat — Linoleic Acid	Polyunsaturated Fat — Alpha-Linole-nic Acid	Predominant Fatty Acids
Coconut	90	7	2	<0.5	Saturated
Palm kernel	82	15	2	<0.5	Saturated
Ghee	65	32	2	<1.0	Saturated
Vanaspati	24	19	3	<0.5	Saturated
Red palm oil (raw)	50	40	9	<0.5	Saturated + Monounsaturated
Palm oil	45	44	10	0.5	" "
Olive	13	76	10	<0.5	Monounsaturated
Groundnut	24	50	25	<0.5	Monounsaturated
Rape/Mustard	8	70	12	1.0	Monounsaturated
Sesame	15	42	42	1.0	Mono and poly-unsaturated
Rice bran	22	41	35	1.5	Mono and poly-unsaturated
Cotton seed	22	25	52	1.0	Polyunsaturated
Corn	12	32	55	1.0	Polyunsaturated
Sunflower	13	27	60	<0.5	Polyunsaturated
Safflower	13	17	70	<0.5	Polyunsaturated
Soya bean	15	27	53	5.0	Polyunsaturated

Table 1.6 Cholesterol Content of Animal Foods

Item	Fat g/100 g	Saturated Fatty Acids g/100 g	Cholesterol mg/100 g
Butter	80	50	250
Ghee	100	65	300
Milk (cow)	4	2	14
Milk (buffalo)	8	4	16
Milk (skimmed)	0.1	–	2
Milk (condensed)	10	6	40
Cream	13	8	40
Cheese	25	15	100
Egg (whole)	11	4	400
Egg yolk	30	9	1120
Chicken without skin	4	1	60
Chicken with skin	18	6	100
Beef	16	8	70
Mutton	13	7	65
Pork	35	13	90
Organ Meats			
Brain	6	2	2000
Heart	5	2	150
Kidney	2	1	370
Liver	9	3	300
Sea Foods	2	0.3	150
Prawn/shrimps			
Fish (lean)	1.5	0.4	45
Fish (fatty)	6	2.5	45

Table 1.7 Cholesterol Counter in Convenient Measures

Item	Quantity	Cholesterol (mg)
Whole milk	1 glass	50
Ice Cream	1 cup	84
Whole egg (or egg yolk)	1 no.	210
Butter	1 tbsp	36
Simmed milk	1 glass	7
Frozen yogurt	1 cup	10
Egg white	1 no.	0
Cream	1 cup	180

1 tbsp (tablespoon)   = 15 ml
1 cup (big)   = 210 ml
1 glass   = 300 ml

2. Asthma

What is Asthma

Asthma is characterized by narrowing of lung airways (bronchi) and excessive production of mucus secretions in the airways. It makes respiration difficult and a feeling of breathlessness and suffocation in chest is felt by the sufferer.

Types of Asthma

There are two types of Asthma:

1. **Bronchial Asthma**—So called because the trouble occurs in the bronchi
2. **Cardiac Asthma**—Here the basic problem lies in the heart and breathlessness is due to heart failure.

The asthma that is normally talked about is bronchial asthma and we shall deal only with this in the present chapter.

Physiological Changes in Asthmatic Attack

During an attack of asthma, following reactions occur in the body:

1. There is a spasm in the muscles of bronchial airways leading to reduced inner diameter of the bronchi (termed as **bronchoconstriction**).
2. The inner lining (mucous membrane) of the bronchi gets swollen, further narrowing the lumen of the bronchi.
3. Secretions are poured out from the swollen mucous lining into the narrowed bronchi and bronchioles.

These changes result in difficulty in breathing, accompanied by a wheezing sound, which is louder during exhalation because then the bronchi get narrower. Expiration demands a continuous muscular effort in order to overcome the added resistance of thick sticky mucus plugging the airways. *The patient may partially accomplish this by exhaling with pressed lips or while whistling, as this builds up the expiratory pressure in the lungs.*

Asthmatic attacks usually occur in the early morning because according to biorhythm of the body it is a sensitive period for lungs and airways. The victim suddenly arouses from his sleep by the attack. He sits up, stoops forward, tightly holds to some object and gasps for breath. The attack subsides after a varying period, either on its own or due to the effects of the medicines administered.

Lungs of Asthma patients are less elastic than those of normal persons and they remain overdistended. The breathing capacity of the lung is decreased leading to disturbed ventilation and improper oxygenation of blood.

Causes of Asthma

1. **Allergy:** Asthma is prominently an allergic disorder. Allergy is an abnormal reaction of the body to a normally harmless substance. Substances like pollens of flowers, spores of fungi, house dust, eggs, fish, wheat, nickel, chromium or milk are harmless to most people, except those who are allergic to them. These are called allergens. The body opposes such an allergen or antigen by producing antibodies.

   When the offending allergen and antibodies react, substances like histamine and serotonin are released into the blood stream. These released substances give rise to various manifestations of allergy like spasm (involuntary contraction) of the muscles of lung airways in case of asthma and other types of symptoms in other cases.

2. **Heredity:** The hereditary factor in Asthma is well recognized, for the disease frequently appears to be passed on from one generation to another within a family. Even

where no positive family history of asthma is detected, there is often a family tendency to some other allergic disorder. Infact what is inherited is allergy and not a particular manifestation of allergy. A parent may have asthma and amongst his sons, one may have eczema and the other sneezing. Similarly a person may have eczema in childhood, develop sneezing when he grows up and then may contract asthma. Asthma, seasonal or perennial sneezing, urticaria (swelling and redness of skin) and eczema are many and different manifestations of one condition called allergy. About 50% of asthma patients give a family history of either asthma or some other form of allergy.

3. **Psychological Causes:** Psychological factors are well recognized in the onset of Asthma. At the psychological levels, suppression of negative emotions such as jealousy, anger, resentment and hatred is often a precipitating cause, as are loneliness, longing for affection, emotional hypersensitivity, fear of rejection and hesitation in life.

Generally the asthmatic is one who has undergone some form of painful rejection or loss early in life which he has been unable to accept subconsciously, even if his conscious mind has come to terms with it. The sufferer feels he is all alone without anyone to depend on, fighting for his very existence as symbolized by his elusive breath.

4. **Infection:** Infection makes an allergy prone individual getting symptoms of allergy. A preexisting sensitivity to specific allergen may become manifest in the presence of infection.

5. **Climate:** Asthma can also arise during changing climatic condition and incidence of attacks is higher in the winter and rainy season in the tropics. The reason is that when cold air strikes your lungs, it constricts the tiny blood vessels which must extract oxygen from the air you breath. The result is reduced oxygen. This is taxing on your bronchial respiratory tubes and your heart, too.

Similarly in humid atmosphere, the amount of water vapour in the air is greatly increased. It lowers the pressure of oxygen in the air which reduces the diffusion of oxygen in the blood calling for more respiratory effort to bring in the same oxygen in the body.

6. **High Altitude:** Going to higher altitudes also becomes the problem for Asthmatic patients. At high altitudes, the atomospheric pressure decreases and concentration of oxygen in the air also reduces resulting in reduced diffusion of oxygen in the body and calling for more respiratory efforts.

7. **Diet and Life Style:** Unhealthy diet and lifestyle also play a role in the genesis of asthma. A low residue, mucus producing diet consisting of excessive refined carbohydrate products like bread and cakes, ghee and oily preparations, milk and milk products is the common culprit. Besides producing mucous, this diet is excessively taxing on the asthmatic's preweakened digestive processes.

Asthma problem can aggravate in those types of occupation and places which are full of pollution, dirt and those allergens which a person is allergic to.

Preliminary Symptoms of Asthmatic Attack

In most asthmatics, there is a sudden onset of cold symptoms —nasal congestion, nasal irritation, bouts of sneezing, indicating that the nasal mucus membrane is becoming swollen and secretry in response to some trigger. As the attack ensues, mucus secretion becomes thick and sticky and a moist cough develops. The chest becomes hyper-expanded and the lungs hyper-inflated. The development, duration and severity of attacks varies between individuals. The attack may develop in minutes or take hours to reach its peak; it may cause minor discomfort and breathlessness or may be severe enough to cause total incapacity and require hospitalization. Death from an asthmatic attack is rare except in elderly people who have other diseases as well.

Treatment of Asthma during Attack

a. Treatment at Home

1. Inhale steam. This will dilate the airways and help in loosening the mucous and its coming out.

2. Drink warm water or any other warm liquid such as soup or lime juice.

3. Put hot water bag on chest and abdomen.

4. Do rigorous massage on the upper and middle back.

5. Lie on your stomach on the bed with chest and head coming out of the bed and stooping towards the floor with the help of hands resting on floor. Have someone thumbing or hacking your back with his hands for a few minutes. This helps to loosen the mucous and allowing it to come out with the help of gravity. It is important to cough out as much mucous as possible. The above technique of removal of cough is known as chest percussion and postural drainage.

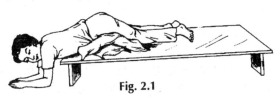

Fig. 2.1

6. Sit in a comfortable position on a chair or stool leaning on a table with your head on a pillow. Now breath in forcibly through one nostril which is more open and force air out through the mouth. Hold breath for a few seconds, then repeat. Make sure that your breathing is abdominal i.e. during inhaling your stomach should come out and during exhalation, it should go in.

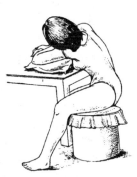

Fig. 2.2

b. **Medical Treatment:** Treatment during an attack consists of:

1. Administering oxygen through nose in case the attack has been very severe and has resulted into a deficiency of oxygen in the blood.

2. Expanding the airways and inhibiting the production of secretions by bronchodilator drugs like Deriphylline, Salbuta-mol (Asthaline), Theophylline, Aminophylline.

Side-effects of these drugs are mainly adverse effect on heart in the form of palpitation. Bronchodilators are given either in the form of tablets or injections or spray in a pressurized aerosol for inhalation.

3. Giving intravenous glucose-saline, if the patient seems dehydrated. If Asthma attack is not adequately controlled by bronchodilators, corticosteriod drugs may have to be given. If there is lung infection, suitable antibiotic drugs also need one to be given.

Long-term Treatment of Asthma

1. **Diet:** An asthmatic's diet should be quite light and balanced. The stomach shouldn't be overloaded with food, especially at dinner. A heavy stomach predisposes one to Asthma attacks.

Food items that are known to produce an allergic reaction or which are known to produce indigestion or flatulence should be strictly avoided. **Mucus forming foods such as rice, potatoes, banana, *urad, rajmah,* ladies finger, sweets, dairy products and refined flour products should be completely avoided.** All chemically treated processed, flavoured and preserved foods should be strictly avoided. Certain other foods like reddish, citrus fruit, curd, cold items are known to precipitate attacks of asthma in persons predisposed to the disease especially when consumed at night. Excessive refined carbohydrates like bread, cakes, pastries and ice-creams, chocolates, oily and ghee preparations should also be avoided.

Similarly, spicy and fried things, chutneys, pickles, sweets and milk products should usually be avoided, especially at dinner. The dinner should be light and should be taken two hours before going to sleep.

Asthmatics should consume seasonal fruits and vegetables in plenty. Asthmatics lose a lot of water through fast and laboured respiration, especially during an attack. Therefore, they should drink water freely. Consumption of alcohol and tobacco (in any form, especially smoking) is strictly prohibited for all asthmatics.

Eating spices such as chilli, pepper, garlic and ginger is advised, especially in colder months when 'Kapha' increases in the body. Fasting is good for Asthma patients. If full fast can't be undertaken, it is a good habit to miss the evening meal and take only hot lemon juice and honey or herbal tea (lemon grass, tulsi, ginger, black pepper).

2. **Breathing Exercises (Pranayama):** Breathing exercises are a boon to asthma patients. Although all yogic pranayama exercises are good for the patient because they all develop respiratory capacity and strengthen and tone up respiratory muscles, however following types of exercises should be specially emphasised.

   a. Blowing up balloons, blowing bubbles, blowing table tennis balls across a table or blowing on a musical instrument (like flute) in order to build up more expiratory pressure and capacity which is so crucial for an asthmatic.

   b. Use of diaphragm and abdominal muscles should be stimulated in preference to chest muscles. In other words, asthmatics need to employ lower chest breathing and decrease upper chest breathing.

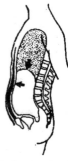 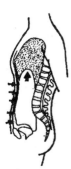

During inhalation, the diaphragm contracts downwards and the abdomen expands

During exhalation, the diaphragm relaxes and the abdomen contracts

Fig. 2.3 Abdominal or Diaphragmatic breathing

This can be practised by putting one hand on abdomen while sitting or lying and then ensuring that during inhalation, abdomen rises and while exhalation, abdomen goes in. Such breathing is especially useful during an attack. Besides, during an attack, the air should be breathed out through a partially open mouth (like whistling).

31

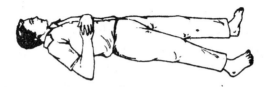

Fig. 2.4 Practising abdominal breathing by putting hands on upper abdomen (above navel)

3. **Aerobic Exercises:** Aerobic exercises (like running, jogging, brisk walking, cycling etc.) should be done upto the limit of panting. This also helps in building up the respiratory capacity.

4. **Neti Kriya:** Neti kriya (nasal cleaning through luke warm salt water) removes obstructions from the nasal passages, facilitates nasal breathing and averts the allergic and hypersensitivity responses mediated through the nasal mucus membrane and its autonomic nervous connections, precipitating bouts of asthma.

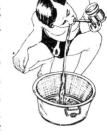

Fig. 2.5 Jal Neti

5. **Removal of Constipation:** Asthmatic should keep his digestive system in order. It is not possible to attain lasting relief or cure in asthmatic in whom constipation remains. He must adhere to a light, simple and well balanced diet. Any gas, acidity in the system irritates mucus lining of airways. Drinking lot of water and doing 'Shankhprakshalan' yogic kriya (see chapter 9) is helpful in removing constipation. At some occasions 'Enema' can be also taken to clean the bowel.

6. **Yogasanas:** All those asanas which improve circulation in chest region and which promote abdominal breathing are particularly good for asthmatic patient e.g.

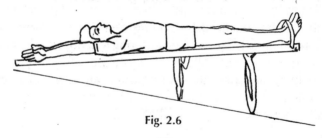

Fig. 2.6

Shashankasana (cat stretch), Sarvangasana, Hastpadasana, Yogmudra. Lying on a slanting board with head down is good for improving circulation in chest region (see Fig. 2.6). But one shouldn't suddenly get up. He should sit and wait for sometimes, before standing up.

7. **Control of Psychological Factors:** As already mentioneu, negative emotions like fear, anxiety, depression, guilt, panic, sudden excitement, anger, to name just a few, can provoke asthma. Mental tension and asthma are closely interlinked. Hence it is necessary to adopt positive mental attitudes about the happenings of life. He must learn to accept whatever comes in life joyfully instead of grumbling. Bringing a sense of calm detachment will go a long way in helping asthma patient. Further, whenever any mental tension appears, he should try to calm down himself by abdominal breathing and lying in Savasana.

General Do's and Don'ts for Asthma Patient

1. Rise early in morning, sunrise is a sensitive period for asthmatics and they should be active at sunrise and not lying down

2. When you get out of bed in the morning, immediately put on a warm covering

3. Bath in warm water in winter. Don't go out right after a bath

4. Avoid direct cold breeze on the face, as this causes a spasm and production of mucus in the sinuses

5. Don't walk barefoot. Keep your feet warm

6. Take morning walk in fresh air

7. At night go to sleep early and at regular hour

8. Have the dinner light and at least two hours before sleeping

9. Keep your house specially the bedroom clean and dust-free. Have no rugs or carpets in your bedroom

10. Have adequate sleep

11. Don't overeat

12. Keep yourself away from smoke, pollution and dust

Chances of Your being a Potential Asthmatic

Consider the following questions

1. Is there a history of asthma in the family?
2. Do you have coughing at the change of season?
3. Do you have bouts of sneezing at the change of season?
4. Do you always have a running nose?
5. Do you often suffer from sore throat?
6. Do you easily get breathless
7. Do you have breathing problems in a strong wind?
8. Do you work/live in a polluted environment?
9. Do you frequently have unexplained skin rashes?

The greater the number of your answers in 'Yes', the greater the chances of your developing asthma.

3. Headache and Migraine

Introduction

Headache is one of the most common of all symptoms afflicting the human race. Headaches may be due to a wide variety of causes such as High Blood Pressure, eye strain, psychological tension, infection of the nose, throat and ears, various tumours and infections inside brain, head injuries, stiffness of neck etc. etc. However, most headaches are functional and are more or less transient i.e. they come today and go tomorrow and not related to any organic changes in the brain.

Strange as it may seem, the brain itself is not sensitive to pain. This means that most headaches are not due to any actual damage within the brain itself. However, any stretching or pressure on the coverings of the brain will most certainly produce a severe pain or headache. Actually in headache, pain is experienced by the person mainly through the blood vessels feeding blood to the brain. Blood vessels supplying blood to the brain are sensitive to pain. Their distension, distortion and inflammation is felt as pain. Anything that affects brain blood supply can cause pain to be registered on the pain receptors in the arteries and veins involved. Therefore in 99% of the headaches, the pain comes from outside the skull. It owes its origin to the tissues lying outside of the skull and under the skin i.e. the muscles and blood vessels of the scalp and neck. The actual source of pain, however, is the end of the pain nerve. Any inflammation within the head, such as occurs in meningitis, will cause extreme pain over the entire head. However, such causes are extremely rare. A tumour growing within the head may press upon the meningeal covering or dura. This causes a severe headache which is usually felt on the side of the head where the tumour is located. Various types of headache are discussed below in detail.

Types of Headache

The types of headache can be summarized into two broad categories:

1. **Headache due to causes outside the brain:** These include (a) Sinusitis (b) Eye strain (c) Toothache (d) Cervical Spondylosis (e) Temporal arteritis (f) Stretching and contraction of the muscles and blood vessels in the neck and scalp (g) Indigestion, Constipation, Acidity.

2. **Headache due to causes inside the brain:** These include brain tumours, bleeding in the space around the brain and High blood pressure.

Below are given the details of these various types of headache:

Tension Headache

Headache due to contraction of the muscles of neck is called tension headache. More than 70% of all headaches are tension headache. You can identify painful areas on the muscles at the back of your neck by running your fingers on any side of the back of neck.

Prolonged psychological tension, sitting in poor posture or sitting in one posture for a long time often seem to produce a spasm of the muscles in the back of the neck. The muscle spasm draws the tissues over the surface of the cranium very tight, so that the pain is felt not only in the back of the neck, but also over the top and front of the head. This is a steady, aching type of pain and usually there is no nausea, vomitting or flashing lights. To avoid such headaches it is important to avoid emotional stress and do neck stretching and rolling exercises whenever you happen to stand or sit in one posture for a long time. Prolonged contraction of eye muscles, scalp muscles and facial muscles can also produce tension headache.

Alcoholic Headache

Many people suffer from a severe headache due to hangover after taking large quantities of alcohol. Alcohol is toxic to the tissues and directly irritates the meninges or coverings of the brain, thus causing pain in the head. The alcohol also dilates the arteries in the brain and this in turn produces a pain like migraine. Naturally the best treatment for this type of headache is to avoid excessive use of alcohol. Also bed rest is advisable till the crisis is over.

Headache due to Acidity/Constipation

It appears to arise from absorbing toxin products from the colon. During constipation, the uneliminated food gets putrefied in the system and releases toxins, gases and acids. These gases and toxins enter the blood and irritate various cells and nerve cells in the head.

Irritation of nerve cells causes headache. A late heavy meal especially during a feast or party causes a severe headache which is accompanied by nausea and vomiting. This is, of course, due to over eating of oily and over cooked food which are indigestible at that time and which result in increased biliousness and hence headache. Various diseases in the body and medications taken also release toxins in the blood which often lead to headache. Similarly toxins in an unclean or chemical environment (e.g. paint, petroleum) inhaled by us during breathing also enter the blood and this can create headache. Further, acidic food taken in excess (e.g. sugar) makes the blood acidic and produces the headache because of irritation of nerve cells by acidity. In this type of headache (also called Toxemic headache) pain is felt normally all over the head region or in some cases just in the frontal region.

Headache due to High Blood Pressure

This headache is due to the increased pressure within the smaller arteries and other blood vessels within the brain. It is usually experienced at the back of head and it is more severe when the person wakes up in the morning.

Sinus Headache

Some of the nasal sinuses lie very close to the brain. Any inflammation within these sinuses may produce a rather severe type of headache. Because of the inflammation of the sinuses, the oxygen level comes down due to obstruction and thus the level of CO_2 increases in the system. This further leads to congestion in the brain tissue which is starved of oxygen and results in a headache. This pain is usually worse when the patient awakens in the morning but generally improves during this day when an erect posture is maintained. It worsens when he shakes his head or gets under strain. This headache is also seen increasing with sunlight and decreasing in the evening when sun sets. Sinusitis is initiated by colds and other respiratory infections which result in congestion of nose and respiratory tract.

Headache due to Eye Strain

Within the eyeball the small ciliary muscles control the shape of the lens of the eye. This enables us to focus our vision on the object we are looking at. Prolonged contraction of these tiny muscles can be a cause of headache due to 'eyestrain'. Also the muscles that move the eye (extraocular muscles) may go into tension, particularly if the muscles controlling one eye are not balanced with those of the other side. This imbalance may cause blurring of vision so that the head may have to be held in a certain position in order to focus the vision. This in turn causes chronic contraction of the muscles of the neck, causing headache.

Further, if the eyes are exposed to a very bright light, a headache may develop lasting 24 to 48 hours possibly due to irritation of the delicate tissues in the eyes. Looking at the sun for only a few seconds may actually burn the retina and cause a severe headache.

Migraine (or Vasular Headache)

Migraine is a throbbing pain usually on one side of the head. It is caused by swelling or dilation of the arteries outside the skull in scalp. Pain is caused by stretching of pain nerve endings ih the arterial wall. This pain is usually associated with nausea, vomiting and increased sensitivity to light and noise. Some persons complain of blind spot in their vision. The pain is severe enough to limit your normal activity.

It is a particular type of severe and recurring head pain. The exact cause is not yet known, though it has been linked with muscular spasm of arteries in the head. The arteries first narrow, then widen, though why they do this is not very clear. One in ten of the adult population is said to suffer from this condition. Before a migraine attack there is often an aura, a warning sign such as flashing lights on zig-zag patterns before the eyes or a tingling feeling in the face or limbs. Then comes the headache—a severe throbbing pain accompanied sometimes with redness and watering of one eye and possibly a running nose. The pain in migraine increases by normal physical works. Common migraine triggers are as follows:

1. Hereditary factors
2. **Environmental Causes:** Heat, cold, bright/glaring light, noise or a humid and cloudy weather can cause migraine in susceptible people.
3. Fatigue, overwork, travel, emotional stress
4. Migraine could also be triggered by either excess or lack of sleep, sometimes by physical stress due to jogging or excitement by sexual activity. Regular exercise helps control migrain but occasional exercise can lead to migraine attack
5. **Food :** Food can cause migrain by three mechanisms–
   a. Decrease in blood glucose levels due to lack of food or fasting
   b. **Tyramine:** It is a chemical compound found in proteins that directly stimulates some cells in the brain. This stimulation constricts the blood vessels of the brain. Foods rich in tyramine are cheese, beer, red wine, chocolate, beef, liver, canned meats, soya sauce, eggs, broad beans, spinach, oranges, figs, prunes, plums, dates, bananas and tomatoes.
   c. Some foods cause allergic reactions. The allergic reaction results in migraine. Common food allergies in migraine are milk, cheese, tea, coffee, orange juice, tomatoes and potatoes.

d. Some people complain of migraine after eating **Chinese food**. This is because Chinese food contains a compound called **monosodium gluconate**. This compound constricts blood vessels of the brain.

e. Apart from this, **the nitrates** and **the nitrites used as colouring agents and as preservatives for some foods may be the cause for headaches.**

f. Smell of paints from freshly painted surfaces can also trigger migraine.

6. **Withdrawal Headache:** People who drink lot of tea, coffee or cola drinks develop headache on sudden withdrawal of caffeine. Reduced intake of caeffine causes distension of blood vessels and therefore headache.

7. **Hormonal Changes:** Decreased oestrogen level in women just before menstruation can trigger a migraine. Women who take contraceptive pills with oestrogen are likely to have very severe migraine.

Neuralgia

Neuralgia is a painful affliction following the course of a nerve or its branches. Trigeminal (5th cranial nerve) neuralgia, whose cause is unknown, is one of the most painful of the neuralgias. Recurring paroxysms of burning pain occur in one side of the face or in the ear and throat as a result of glossopharyngeal neuralgia. While the latter can be cured by cutting the glossopharyngeal nerve, in the former case the trigeminal nerve inside the skull is cut to provide permanent relief.

Temporal Arteritis

Temple is the region between and just above your eyes and ears. The artery which runs across the temple on both sides is called **temporal artery.** Rarely, there is inflammation of the tissues inside this artery. This condition is called temporal arteritis. It is not a common disease but if not treated, can cause blindness almost overnight. It can also reduce blood supply to part of the brain and result in stroke.

Temporal arteritis is mainly observed in people above fifty years. Any new headache in the temple in elderly people should be investigated for temporal arteritis. The artery is sometimes prominent and painful to touch. If the doctor suspects temporal arteritis, he will ask you to undertake a blood test called the ESR (Erythrocyte Sedimentation Rate). An ESR reading more than 50 mm in first one hour indicates temporal arteritis. The doctor may also remove a small piece of the artery and examine it under microscope. This is called biopsy and is the confirmative test for temporal arteritis. Steroids are the only medicines recommended for treatment of temporal arteritis.

Headache due to Tuberculoma

A tumour, abscess or chronic inflammatory mass such as the 'Tuberculoma' are the common causes of increased pressure of the brain. They may not cause headaches in the early stages. Very often the headache is observed only after more serious complications such as paralysis. Any tumour that grows inside the skull puts pressure on the brain at the site of its growth. It also stops the outflow of the cerebrospinal fluid and therefore raises pressure within the skull. A rise in the pressure causes dull persistant headaches.

Headache due to Meningitis

Meningitis is the infection of the loose coverings of the brain called the 'meninges'. The brain floats in a fluid called the 'Cerebro spinal fluid'. This fluid supports the brain and protects it from shocks. Sometimes the meninges get infected and start producing pus. The pus is full of bacteria. It directly enters the cerebro spinal fluid in which the brain floats. The bacteria and viruses come in direct contact with the brain and infect it very quickly. The common symptoms of meningitis are fever, headache, stiffness of the neck and vomiting. The patient can't tolerate light and soon becomes drowsy or unconscious. Anyone who has fever and stiff neck should be rushed to a major hospital immediately. The faster the treatment, greater are the chances of recovery. Delayed treatment often results in death.

Site of Pain for Various Causes of Headache

S.No.	Site of pain	Figure	Type of Headache
1.	Front of the head		Tension headache Toothache Sinusitis
2.	Sides of the head		Tension headache Migraine Temporal arteritis
3.	Middle or all over		Tension headache Tumour

4.	Back of the head and/or neck		Tension headache
			Meningitis
			Subarachnoid
			   haemorrhage
			Cervical
			   spondylosis
			Hypertension

5.	Around/above the eyes		Tension headache Migraine Cluster headache

Some Generalised Causes
of Headache

- **Diet:** Excessive intake of heavy and sour articles and greens, and drinking very cold water are common causes of headache. Poor digestion of food results in putrefaction of food inside the intestines also results in headache.

- **Life-style:** Suppression of natural desires, sleeping during the day time, inadequate sleep at night, alcohol intake, talking very loudly, exposure to cold weather.

- Excess of sexual act also causes headache.

- **Environment:** Unpleasant smell, facing head-winds, and exposure to dust, smoke, cold and heat can also cause headache.

- **Psychological:** Psychological stress, excessive worry or suppression of tears can lead to headache.

- **Season:** Some people have headache when there is abnormality in normal climate or season, or just before the onset of rains.

- **Injury:** Any injury to the head, irrespective of its severity, can cause headache.

Treatment of Headache

1. Headache Due to Indigestion

The following measures will prevent gas formation due to indigestion and thereby prevent headache.

    a. **Drinking at least eight to ten glasses of water every day:** You should drink one glass of water every two hours. You should also drink three to four glasses of water on empty stomach as soon as you get up. This helps to activate your bowel movements.

    b. **Passing stools every morning and evening:** You should train your body to evacuate twice a day. This will prevent formation of gases from undigested food.

    c. **Abdominal pack:** Three hours after every dinner, keep a cloth dipped in cold water on the abdomen for twenty minutes. This abdominal pack will increase blood circulation of various organs in your abdomen. Increased circulation improves digestion.

d. **Enema:** A warm water enema is recommended if you suffer from constipation. You should evacuate after five to ten minutes of taking the enema. In case it is not possible to take enema, then take some ayurvedic powder like 'Kabzahara' (Baidyanath) or Kabzola (M/s Tabex Pharma) in the night with hot water. It will clear your bowels in the morning.

2. Treatment of Tension Headache

Physical and mental stress results in tightening of muscles of the head and neck. This tightening results in the headache. The following measures help relax your head and neck muscles:

- Stretching of the neck and shoulders relieves pain.

- Massaging the head, neck and shoulders. Some of the massaging actions on neck and shoulders for removing their stiffness are shown in Figs. 5.5 and 5.6. Moving acupressure roller on the back of your neck starting from the upper back upto base of scale also relaxes your stiff neck as shown in following figure.

- Keep a hot water bag or heating pad on the neck. Heat increases the blood circulation and therefore relaxes the muscles.

- Pouring hot and cold water on the neck alternately also results in increased blood circulation. This results in relaxation of muscles.

- Keeping your backbone in contact with cold water in a special spinal bath tub for thirty minutes relaxes the mind. A relaxed mind helps control the headaches.

3. Headache Caused due to Cold, Sinus and other Upper Respiratory Infection

Colds and other respiratory infections result in congestion of the nose and respiratory tract. This congestion can cause headache. The following measures are recommended for reducing the congestion of the respiratory tract:

a. **Hot Foot Bath:** In this bath, you should keep your legs up to knees in a bucket of hot water. Your body should be covered with a blanket to prevent loss of body heat. The head should be covered with a cold cloth. A hot foot bath for five to twenty minutes helps control the headaches in three ways: (a) it increases bowel movements; (b) relieves congestion due to cold and (c) constricts dilated blood vessels of the brain. It is important to remember that you should drink at least one glass of water before taking this bath.

b. **Steam Inhalation:** Inhaling steam increases blood circulation of the head and the respiratory organs. It also opens up the nasal passages. Increased blood circulation and open nasal passages reduce the congestion.

c. **Steam Bath:** In this bath, the Nature Cure doctor will ask you to sit in a special cabinet for ten to twenty minutes. This will result in a lot of sweating. Increased sweating removes waste matter in your body. You should have a cold water bath immediately after the steam bath. Alternative steam and cold bath increases blood circulation. You should drink one or two glasses of cold water before taking the steam bath and cover your head with a cold towel.

Note: Pregnant women, and those with heart diseases or high blood pressure should not take this bath. It is important to remember that if you feel tired or uncomfortable during the bath, you should come out of the steam cabinet immediately and drink cold water.

4. Headache Due to Eye Strain

If headache is due to eye strain, apply cold compress on the eyes. It has a wonderful effect.

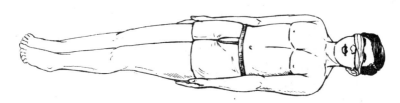

Fig. 3.1

You can also relax your eyes by pinching the flesh of your eyebrows and by massaging around the eye socket in a circular motion.

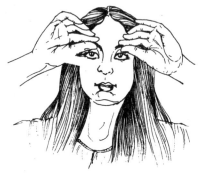

Fig. 3.2

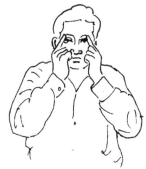

Fig. 3.3 Massaging around eye socket

5. Treatment for Migraine Headache

The following measures should be taken as soon as you get migraine. These measures reduce distention of the blood vessels of the brain.

- Vomiting after taking four to five glasses of luke warm water with salt.
- Hot foot bath.
- Enema to clear clogged bowels.
- Sip warm water bit by bit. It sometimes helps in bringing the headache down. You can also take hot honey water or vegetable soups.
- Massage head by various techniques (see details later).
- Apply cold pack on the head (specially on temples and back of the head) and sleep for a while in a dark room. Cold compress will constrict distended blood vessels of the brain. Sleeping in a dark room will help you relax.

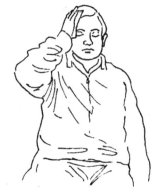

Fig. 3.4 Cold Pack on temples

46

- Apply Badam Roghan or any other Ayurvedic pain relieving oil on your forehead and massage it.

Diet for Prevention of Headache

One should take high fibre diet and avoid refined, processed and canned foods. High fibre diet improves bowel movements and helps complete evacuation of stools. Thus there will be no acid and gas formation in the digestive system. You should eat regular meals consisting of whole cereals, nuts, fruits, leafy vegetables, legumes and tubers. Avoid milk and milk products too much as they can trigger migraine headaches. Citrous fruits and their juices remove toxins from the body. Removal of toxins often helps control the headaches. However, you should avoid citrous fruits during migraine attacks. All other foods which predispose one to migraine attack e.g. Tyramine or some other allergic foods should be avoided and during the attack shouldn't be taken at all. Such foods are mentioned in this chapter where migraine headache is explained.

Common Misconceptions and Their Clarifications about Headache

S. No.	Misconception	Clarification
1.	People with recurrent headaches have psychological problems	This is not True. Headaches occur due to some bio-chemical changes in the brain. Psychological stress results in release of chemical substances in the brain. These substances can lead to headaches. However, psychological problems usually do not cause headaches.
2.	There is no cure of recurrent headaches and people have to learn to live with the pain.	Headaches may not be cured forever. Most people can reduce pain and the disability of headaches through proper medical care, changes in the life styles and relaxation techniques.

Contd...

S. No.	Misconception	Clarification
3.	Recurrent headaches are not serious. They do not require any treatment.	Most headaches do not cause death but adversely affect the quality of life. People need to manage frequent episodes of headaches to prevent strain on the family life and career opportunities.
4.	The only treatment for headaches is taking medicines during pain.	Medicines can reduce the pain during an episode of headache but they cannot always prevent recurrent headaches. It is necessary to adopt healthy life-styles for managing the headaches.
5.	More frequent the headaches, more likely are the chances of serious brain disorders.	This is never true. In fact the opposite is true. The biggest threat is from sudden, severe and unusual headaches that are dangerous and indicate some serious diseases.
6.	All severe headaches are called migraine.	This is not always true. Migraine is a specific disease of the nervous system which produces one-sided headache, and is accompanied by other symptoms also.
7.	High Blood pressure is one of the common causes of headaches.	This is not true. Very few people with high blood pressure complain of recurrent headaches.
8.	All headaches are very serious and may cause brain disorder.	Serious headaches are only 1% of all headaches and one should not worry about developing serious diseases such as brain tumor.

Miscellaneous Massage and Acupressure Treatments for Headache/Migraine

1. Press the head with more emphasis on front and back portion of head (see Fig. 3.5).

2. Press with both thumbs into the base of your skull on the hollows on either side of centre line a few times. You can also press these points with a two ball arrangement as shown in the Fig. 3.7.

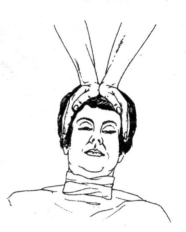

Fig. 3.5

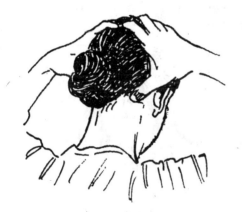

Fig. 3.6

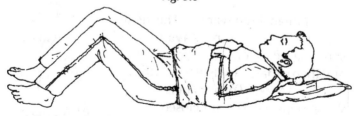

Fig. 3.7 Double ball of shape (OO) connected together by making holes in them and placed below base of skull as shown

3. Pull the hair of your head on all sides until your scalp tingles, with special emphasis near back of head and near temples.

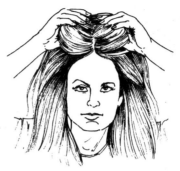

Fig. 3.8

4. Massage and rub your head with the tips of your fingers with special emphasis on the back of your head and area around the temples.

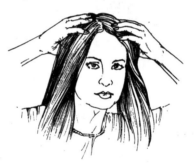

Fig. 3.9

5. Do 'Gunjan Pranayama'. The healing vibrations of this pranayama has a soothing effect on head. Inhale deeply and then exhale slowly through the nose making the sound of humming from your throat. Lips will remain closed.

6. Place your thumbs at the centre of the forehead of the patient just above the brows, anchoring your hands on the sides

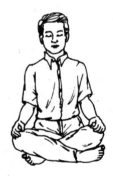

Fig. 3.10

of the head. Moving up a strip at a time, draw your thumbs apart slowly, coming out over the hair and off the sides of the head. Cover the whole forehead in this way, travelling up as far as the hairline. Patient can also do this massage himself by using fore and middle fingers of both the hands.

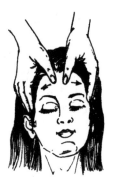

7. Press the points at the inner corners of the eye sockets for 3-5 seconds with your thumb and index finger.

Fig. 3.11

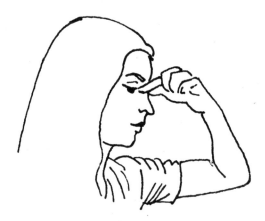

Fig. 3.12

8. Press the points just outside the bony ridge at the outer end of each eyebrow. Press and release a few times.

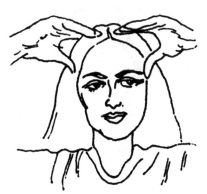

Fig. 3.13

9. With your fingers resting on your head use your thumbs to massage your temples in a series of small circles.

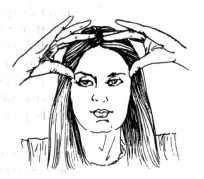

Fig. 3.14

10. With your fingers on your head, massage the inner and outer side of ears with your thumbs in continuous movement.

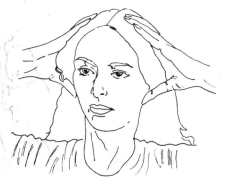

Fig. 3.15

11. Pull your earlobes down a few times.

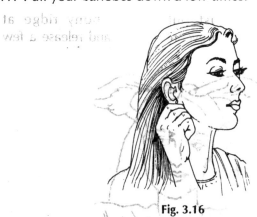

Fig. 3.16

Similarly pull your ears on the sides and in upward direction.

12. Insert the tip of your forefinger inside the ear and vigorously shake it.

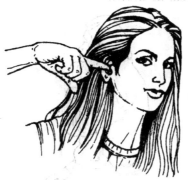

Fig. 3.17

13. Massage the sides of your head using your forefinger kept vertically. Start from the inner edge of ear and reach upto the outer edge of eye socket, massaging the temples.

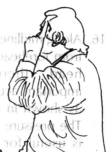

Fig. 3.18

14. Massage the ears by your thumb and forefinger moving up from the lobes to the top of ears covering the whole ear.

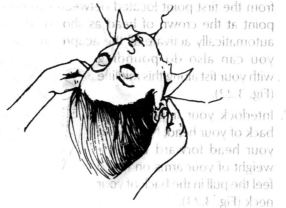

Fig. 3.19

15. Vigorously rub and shake the hard cartilage on the inner side of the ear as shown.

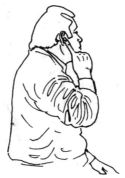

Fig. 3.20

16. Along midline of head starting from forehead upto crown of head, there are many important acupressure points as shown in adjacent figure. The pressure on these points is useful for alleviating the headache.

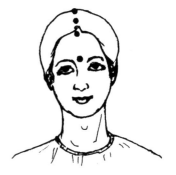

Fig. 3.21

Instead of giving individual pressure, you can also rub the tip of your forefinger along this midline starting from the first point located between eyebrows to the last point at the crown of head as shown. This massage will automatically activate all the acupressure points. Similarly you can also do pounding with your fist along this midline (Fig. 3.22).

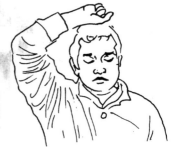

17. Interlock your fingers at the back of your head. Now bend your head forward with the weight of your arms on it and feel the pull in the back of your neck (Fig. 3.23).

Fig. 3.22

In this position (called 'Chin lock' in Yoga), the carotid arteries supplying blood to the brain are compressed which result in fading of nerve impulses in the brain producing a condition akin to anaesthesia and therefore less pain is experienced.

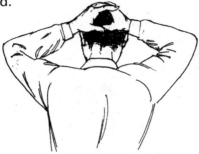

Fig. 3.23

18. Rub the hair brush along your eyebrows upto temple area.

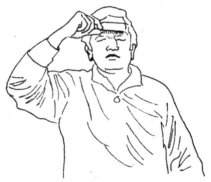

Fig. 3.24

19. Rub the hair brush at the base of skull on the back of head.

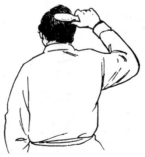

Fig. 3.25

55

20. Press and massage the 'Hoku' point located in the fleshy web between the thumb and forefinger. It is one of the most important points for pain relief in the body.

21. Give Reiki on the temples by putting one hand on left temple and one hand on right temple.

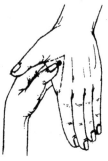

Fig. 3.26

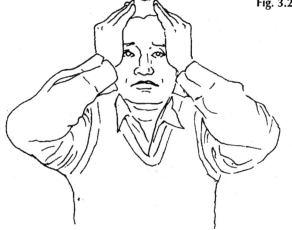

Fig. 3.27

Reiki on the temples can also be given while lying on side as shown in the following figure.

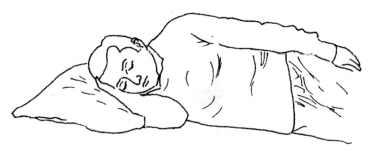

Fig. 3.27 A

22. Give Reiki on the back of head by putting one hand over the other. While lying, it is a very comfortable position to give Reiki to the back of head.

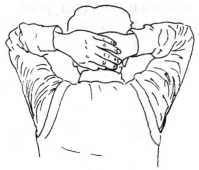

Fig. 3.28

23. Give Reiki to the front of head by placing hands there.

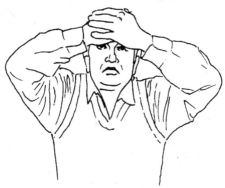

Fig. 3.28A

Reiki to the front of head can also be given more conveniently by lying in prone position as shown in the following figure.

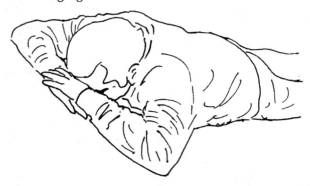

Fig. 3.28 B. Hands to be kept one over the other with palms down, forehead to be kept on back side of hands and chin resting on ground.

24. Tie a cloth piece tightly around your head passing through your temples, forehead and back of head.

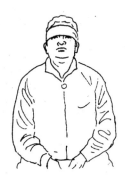

Fig. 3.29

25. Rub or press the tips of fingers and tips of toes with more emphasis on thumb and on big toe. These acupressure points are connected with head.

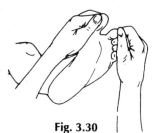

Fig. 3.30

26. Rub hair brush along the dotted line form top of ear to crown of head as shown in the figure.

27. For instant relief of headache/migraine put rubber band tightly on the first joint of all fingers of hands and all toes of feet for 3–5 minutes and then remove before the fingers become blue. Then after 5 minutes continue the same treatment. Cloth pins/clips can also be used in place of rubber bands.

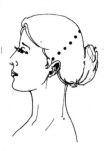

Fig. 3.31

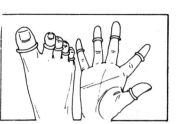
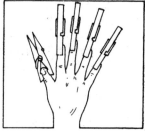

Figs. 3.32 & 3.33

28. Interlock your fingers at the back of your head. Bend your head backwards, at the same time prevent it from doing so by the pressure of your hands. Release the pressure after a few seconds. Do it a few times. It will relax the tense neck muscles at the back. See Fig. 5.8.2 in chapter 5 in ⋅this regard.

29. Press and massage the acupressure points as shown in the figure by forefinger in the form of circling. Exact location of the points can be obtained by you by feeling of tenderness/sensitivity and pain on these points by applying pressure (points just above the ear are approx. at 1/2" interval).

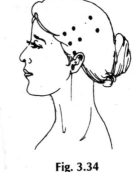

Fig. 3.34

30. Apply acupressure rollers at the base of skull as shown in following figures. Base of the skull is very effective area for alleviating headache.

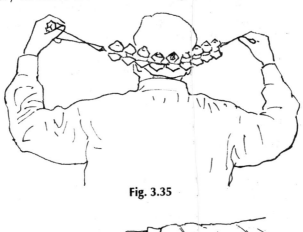

Fig. 3.35

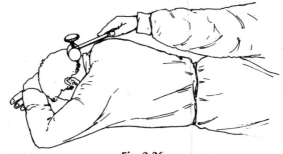

Fig. 3.36

Miscellaneous Nature-cure Treatments for Headache/Migraine

1. Do local pranic sweeping of temple area, front head and back of the head by moving your cupped hand swiftly back and forth a few times over the concerned area and then flicking it in the empty space visualizing that this diseased energy is thrown in cosmos. This process can be repeated many times in one cycle and then several cycles can be done in a day.

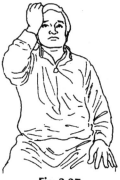
Fig. 3.37

(For more details about the theory and practice of pranic sweeping, please refer my book 'Healing through Reiki'.)

2. If headache is due to hot weather, then breathe from your left nostril by closing your right nostril. Breathing from left nostril increases coolness in the body and helps in reducing such headache. By sleeping on right side (i.e. left hand towards the ceiling) your left nostril tends to open automatically. So you can sleep on your right side. In yoga terminology this is called shifting Swara to the Chandra Nadi (left nostril breathing). Similarly, if headache is due to cold, then breathe from your right nostril by closing left nostril.

3. Put some drops of mustard oil or 'ghee' in that nostril on which side headache is occurring and inhale so that it goes inside up to the mouth.

4. Sometimes headache occurs due to electrolyte imbalance in the body specially when you move a lot in the hot sun. During such situations, you should take some electrolyte like 'Electral' to maintain balance of fluid, salt and sugar in the body.

5. Give Reiki to liver by placing your hands there. It energises the liver and liver removes toxins from the blood more efficiently which sometimes results in reduction of headache.

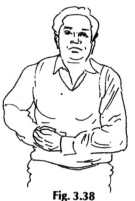
Fig. 3.38

6. Press carotid arteries in the neck (located on both sides of Adam's apple) intermittently. This reduces the blood flow in the brain and hence reduces the headache.

7. Induce sneezing by snuff.

8. While lying on the back in the corpse pose, tie a piece of cloth tightly around each bicep muscle above the elbow (middle of the upper arm). If headache is on one side, then tie the piece of cloth on that arm. This technique is said to give relief in 5-10 minutes itself.

9. Drink lukewarm salted water through nose. Drink lukewarm milk through nose (in summer, cold water without salt and cold milk can be used).

10. Do nadi-shodhan pranayama.

11. Do 'kunjal' kriya if you feel sensation of vomiting due to contents of food lying in stomach.

12. Take out tongue beyond teeth by half an inch and press between teeth. Apply 'Gyan Mudra' by joining tip of index finger with the thumb.

13. Press roof of mouth (hard palate) with the thumb (that portion to which side you are experiencing the headache).

14. Apply mustard oil on navel, ears, sole of the foot and nose specially if headache is due to cold.

15. Apply blue coloured coconut oil on the forehead and temples (Blue oil is prepared after putting coconut oil in blue coloured bottle and placing this bottle in sun for some days so that oil gets charged with blue colour of sun). You can also apply any other ayurvedic pain relieving balm or oil on head.

Useful Information for Migraine Sufferers

(A) List of Migraine Triggerers

1. **Eye strain** due to continuous staring at work place or due to reading in bad light and wrong posture.

2. **Extremes of heat** due to overexposure in hot sun.

3. **Extremes of sound** due to being in constant high level traffic working in noisy environment.

4. Looking at bright and glaring lights.

5. **Extremes of cold:** Moving in highly cold weather and cold winds.

6. **Carbon monoxide:** Remaining in polluted environment e.g. road pollutions industrial pollution which generate large amount of Co.

7. **Chemical fumes and certain smells:** volatile solvents in paints, paint removers, spot removers, gasoline and certain glues.

8. **Poisonous Chemicals:** Working with or being in the vicinity of poisonous chemicals like lead, isocyanides, organic reagents, pesticides, insecticides etc.

9. **Certain Foods:** As listed in the next table. It has been noted that these foods only intensify the headache which has already started but don't usually initiate headache if the person is eating them in the normal healthy condition.

10. **Stress:**

11. **Colouring agents, artificial sweetners, preservatives in foods**

12. **Hormonal fluctuations in women especially before menstrual period:**

(B) List of Foods to be avoided during Migraine Attack

1. Chocolate and chocolate drinks

2. Cheese

3. Acid and Citrus fruits (Lemon, Lime, Orange, Mosambi, Malta, Black Grapes, Grape fruit, Plum, Tomato, Amla, Imli)

4. Caffeine (Coffee, Soft drinks, Tea)

5. Alcohal

6. Sugar

7. Salt

8. Fermented foods (Soya sauce, Idli, Dosa, Dokhlas, Kulchas, Bhaturas, Naans, Bread, Doughnut)

9. Onion

10. Garlic

11. Ice or Ice cold water
12. Vinegar (सिरका)
13. Nuts (specially peanuts)
14. Smoked foods
15. Pickled foods
16. Chinese foods (as they contain Monosodium Glutamate)
17. Processed Meat (as hot dogs, has salami and many other sausages)
18. Sodium Nitrates and Nitrites (used as colouring agents and preservatives in foods)
19. Certain fruits e.g. Bananas, Papayas, Avocado, Pineapple
20. Some Dried fruits such as fig, Raisin, dates, prunes
21. Some dairy products e.g. curd, buttermilk, sour cream
22. Smoking
23. Fats and fried foods
24. Some vegetables like spinach, broad beans, pumpkin, peas
25. Eggs
26. Ice cream
27. Cookies and cakes made with yeast

4. Diabetes

What is Diabetes?

D iabetes is a metabolic disorder which is caused by the deficiency of the hormone Insulin or the inability of body cells to use the available insulin. Insulin is produced in the pancreas. Insulin helps to oxidise glucose in the body in order to release energy. With insufficient Insulin, the glucose accumulates in the blood, causing the symptoms of Diabetes.

Mechanism of Diabetes

The carbohydrates in our food are finally digested in intestine. The end products of carbohydrate digestion are sugars (chiefly glucose). This glucose is absorbed through the mucous membrane of intestines to enter the blood stream. Thus the concentration of glucose in the blood rises. Insulin (from Pancreas) makes this glucose available to each and every cell of the body which uses it as a fuel to generate heat and energy. Insulin is essential for glucose fuel to gain entry into the cellular engine. If the amount of glucose in the blood is greater than cellular requirements, insulin converts it into glycogen which is stored in the liver. Insulin is also concerned with the conversion of excess glucose into fat by the liver which is then stored into adipose tissues.

After taking food, the concentration of glucose in the blood rises. Insulin prevents the glucose concentration from rising above normal or physiological limit. Thus the most important and obvious function of insulin is to control the concentration of glucose in the blood.

If insulin is absent or inadequate, the glucose in the blood can't enter various body cells and also can't be converted into glycogen. Consequently blood glucose level rises. When this blood passes through kidneys, excess sugar (beyond capacity of kidneys to reabsorb) spills into urine.

Normally the nutritional requirements of body cells are met by glucose but when due to deficiency of insulin or due to resistance of cells to insulin, glucose can't enter the cells, cellular starvation starts. To supply nutrition to the starving cells, the body starts disintegrating stored fats and proteins, *which is why body of diabetic patient becomes weak and weight reduces.*

Insulin is also concerned with the metabolism of dietary fats and proteins. The end products of fat digestion are fatty acids. Insulin converts these fatty acids again into fat which is then stored in adipose tissue. Similarly insulin is also essential for protein synthesis in the body. If there is a deficiency of insulin, proteins lost due to wear and tear can't be replaced. Again insulin prevents conversion of stored fat and protein for meeting energy requirements of the body till sugar and stored glycogen are available to meet energy needs.

Types of Diabetes

Most cases of Diabetes are due to two major types, Insulin-dependent Diabetes Mellitus (IDDM) also known as Juvenile Diabetes and Non-insulin-dependent Diabetes Mellitus (NIDDM). IDDM is due to relative or absolute deficiency of insulin. NIDDM is due to inability or resistance of body cells to use the available insulin. The differences between the two are given below.

IDDM

- More common in childhood and young adulthood
- Patients are underweight
- Patients are prone to frequent infections
- Patients exhibit a marked deficiency of insulin
- Patients require lifelong insulin support
- Complications like Diabetic coma are common if insulin is missed
- Accounts for 3–7% of diabetic cases.

NIDDM

- More common in later life, generally after 40 years
- Frequently associated with obesity
- Generally asymptomatic
- Mostly Hereditary
- Treated usually with diet control, exercise and oral drugs when needed
- Diabetic coma is rare
- Accounts for about 90–95% of diabetic cases.

Symptoms of Diabetes

1. Dryness of mouth and excessive thirst
2. Excessive hunger
3. Excessive and frequent urination
4. Weight loss
5. Feeling of exhaustion and weakness
6. Blurring of vision
7. Easy susceptibility to infections of skin, gums and respiratory system
8. Wound infections and delayed healing
9. Sexual debility
10. Lack of concentration and mental fatigue.

Causes of Diabetes

1. **Heredity**
   - If both parents are diabetic, the chances of an individual developing Diabetes are almost 100%
   - If one parent is Diabetic, the chances of the offspring developing Diabetes are about 50%
   - If a close blood relative has diabetes, the risk of an individual developing the disease is about 25%.
2. **Obesity and over-nutrition** are directly related to a higher risk of developing Diabetes. This is because it is found that obesity and more fat intake interfere with proper

functioning of insulin and fat people require greater level of insulin to achieve the same benefit.

3. **Lack of exercise** and the general physical inactivity is also a factor for developing Diabetes.

4. **Tension, anxiety and stress** can precipitate Diabetes in those who have a genetic predisposition to the disease.

5. **Some drugs** including those of the cortisone group can increase the blood sugar and thus may reveal pre-existing Diabetes.

6. **Incorrect dietary habits**—The incidence of diabetes varies directly with the consumption of processed, refined and junk foods e.g. biscuits, bread, cakes, chocolates, pudding, icecream along with over eating.

The body has to produce more digestive juices and insulin to digest excessive food. Under the pressure of excessive work load, the pancreas gland weakens and ultimately breaks down leading to diabetes.

Diabetic Coma or Unconsciousness (Hyperglycemia and Hypoglycemia)

Diabetic coma is commonly seen in Juvenile Diabetes (in child and young persons) but is uncommon in grown up patients. This type of unconsciousness ensues when the concentration of glucose in the blood rises much above the normal **(Hyperglycemia)**. The disintegration of stored fat inside the body is commensurate with the amount of glucose in the blood. The end products of fat disintegration are ketone bodies which due to their acidic nature, make the blood acidic. This acidified blood affects the brain. At first it leads to drowsiness and lethargy and then gradually to diabetic coma. The body tries to get rid of these harmful ketone bodies by producing more and more urine. This however results in a reduction in the fluid content of the body. So the concentration of ketone bodies increases. Thus a vicious circle starts.

A diabetic may also become unconscious when the concentration of glucose in the blood drops much below normal **(Hypoglycemia)**. However, such unconsciousness happens rapidly, while unconsciousness due to excessive glucose and ketosis is a slowly developing condition. Patient experiences various symptoms of uneasiness (e.g. acute thirst, dryness of mouth, weakness, headache, nausea, vomiting, profuse urination etc.) before diabetic coma due to hyperglycemia occurs.

Long Term Complications of Diabetes

In the long run, diabetes ruins almost every system of the body. Complications of the nervous system give rise to distorted sensations, inefficiency of the urinary bladder and sexual debility.

Complications of the heart and blood vessels result in the hardening and narrowing of the arteries (atherosclerosis), high B.P and cronic heart disease. The incidence of heart attacks is about 5-6 times higher in diabetics than in healthy persons.

Diabetes damages the retina of the eyes. This results in gradual loss of vision. Cataract, too, occurs at an early age in diabetics.

Complications of the respiratory system result in an increased susceptibility to infectious diseases of the lungs like T.B.

Diabetes has undesirable effects on the digestive system. Nausea/Vomitting, diarrhoea and gall-stones are more common in diabetics.

Diagnosis and Tests for Diabetes

i. **Benedict's Test:** Usually the Benedict test for detection of urine sugar is done in the laboratory. The method is as follows:

    To 5 c.c. (teaspoonful) of Benedict's Qualitative solution in a test tube, add 8 drops of urine. Boil for 5 minutes, then shake it and allow it to cool. If the contents remain clear in colour, the urine is sugar free. An opaque greenish precipitate indicates 1/2% of sugar, yellow sediment about 1% and red to reddish brown (brick red) sediment more than 2%.

ii. **Clini Test:** Clinitest tablets are available in the market. First a mixture of 5 drops of urine and 10 drops of water is taken in a test tube. A clinitest tablet when dropped in the test tube makes the mixture boil on its own. The hot mixture gradually changes colour. A colour chart provided with the tablets can be used to match the colour of urine and thus ascertain the amount of sugar present.

iii. **Glucose Oxidase Test:** Paper or plastic strips called diastix or tes-tape are available in the market. A colour chart is provided along with the strips. While passing urine two hours after a meal, the person has to hold a tes-tape or a diastix strip in the urine stream for a few moments. The strip changes colour on coming in contact with the urine. This colour is matched with the colours in the chart to determine the amount of sugar in the urine.

iv. **Glucose Tolerance Test (GTT):** This is the most commonly used test to detect blood and urine sugar and thereby ascertain the metabolism of dietary carbohydrates in the body. Blood and urine sugar in both fasting as well as after taking glucose is determined in this test.

Blood Sugar Permissible Limits

Category of Person	Blood Glucose Concentration (in mg%)		
	Fasting Value	Maximum Value	Value 2 hours after Consuming Glucose
Normal	Less than 120	Less than 160	Less than 120
Early Diabetes	120 to 140	160 to 180	120 to 140
Established Diabetes	More than 140	200 or more	More than 140

Treatment of Diabetes

A. **Diet Control:** Diet is the single most important factor for controlling diabetes. If faulty dietary habits are not given up, drug or any other treatments will be of little value. In fact, for obese diabetic, dietary change assumes all the more significance.

For diabetic patient, food containing a large quantity of sugar such as sweets, pastries, ice cream, syrup, honey, cake etc. should be avoided. Also foods rich in starch, such as bread, potatoes and rice should be used in limited quantities. The diabetics have a limited ability to utilize carbohydrates. Increased blood sugar, leakage of sugar in urine and faulty fat metabolism with ketosis result when this ability is overtaxed. Hence concentrated sources of quickly absorbable carbohydrates like sugars etc. should be avoided and pure refined starches should be limited as much as possible. Saturated fats should be avoided if vascular complications have set in. Total amount of calories consumed is the mainstay of adequate dietary control. We can summarise the foods for a diabetic patient in the following manner:

i. **Foods to be Totally Avoided:** All concentrated sources of sugar such as sugar, glucose, jam, chocolates, sweets, sweet drinks, sweetened milk, canned fruits, sweet biscuits, cake, pie, pudding, peppermint and alcohol.

ii. **Foods to be Taken in Limited Quantity:** Cereals, pulses, potatoes, peas, dry fruits, cheese, milk, butter, ghee, oil, meat, eggs, fish, curd.

iii. **Foods That can be Taken Freely:** Most fruits, vegetables, drinks (tea, coffee etc. sweetened with saccharine).

iv. **Special Medicinal Foods:** Certain foods like Bitter gourd (Karela), Black berry (Jamun), 'Trifla', Fenugreek (Methi), Garlic and 'Neem' are considered natural medicinal foods for controlling diabetes. Hence patients of diabetes should consume them often.

v. **Fibre Foods:** Fibres lower the rate of glucose absorption from the gut and thereby lowers glucose level in the blood and therefore it aids in treating diabetes. Fibre helps in reducing insulin dosage administered to the diabetic patient. For fibres take whole grain cereals and pulses alongwith fruits and vegetables.

In addition following practical suggestions will be useful regarding diet for diabetic patients:

1. Diabetics should take more number of smaller meals scattered over the day rather than taking few heavy

concentrated meals so that the blood sugar level doesn't shoot up suddenly as the smaller amount of insulin (or that injected as a medicine) is insufficient to metabolize large amount of blood sugar.

2. Diabetics should avoid fasting and missing their meals to prevent low blood sugar. Even if you don't have appetite, don't abstain from food. Have light food at regular intervals.

3. While on a tour, keep fruits like apples, oranges or sweet limes to prevent low blood sugar.

4. In sweetening agent, saccharine is more preferable to sugar. Although it is sweeter than sugar but it has no calorie content.

5. Maintain your meal timings properly to maintain blood sugar at normal levels all the time.

6. Have variety in your food so that all necessary vitamins, minerals and other nutrients reach to body to keep it fit.

7. Spices can be taken by a diabetic as they possess no calorific value. However, restrict the use of salt.

8. The diabetic should increase his awareness about the disease—how body controls blood sugar, the effects of insulin and other drugs, and the effect of exercise, different foods and other diseases in body.

9. Make sure that friends and associates know that you are diabetic and understand that you cannot take irregular meals or drinks.

10. Avoid operating machinery or driving unless you have eaten in the previous two hours.

11. Children and those particularly prone to hypoglycaemic attacks should carry a card giving details of their condition and instruction for treatment in an emergency.

B. Exercises: Exercise helps the diabetics in many ways. Exercise increases the receptivity of muscles to insulin and greater amount of glucose will be transferred from the blood stream to the muscles by the same amount of insulin. Further during exercise more oxygen is sent to pancreas and thus pancreas is stimulated to function better.

Physical activity will burn blood sugar and lower its level. In the body, glucose can't be metabolized without oxygen.

Exercise provides lot of oxygen to metabolize the sugar. With consistent physical activity, the ability of cells to respond to insulin gradually increases.

There are other indirect good effects of exercise on a diabetic e.g. it reduces triglycerides and LDL cholesterol in the blood. Further, it decreases extra fat which (obesity) is one of the important contributing factors in diabetes.

Isometric exercises involving lifting of weights etc. are not recommended. Aerobic exercises like walking, cycling, swimming are more useful. However, when the blood sugar level is very high and pulse rate becomes very high even in little exertion, exercise should be planned in consultation with a medical expert.

C. **Medicines:** Two types of medicines are used in diabetes.

   i. Oral antidiabetic drugs

   ii. **Insulin injections:** The type and dosage of these medicines has to be determined by an expert physician taking into account the condition of the patient.

D. **Acupressure:** There are acupressure points in palms and soles of the leg corresponding to pancreas as shown in the following figure. Pressing these points regularly and frequently will activate pancreas and gradually it will start functioning better. These acupressure or reflex points are like switches or buttons. When you press them, current or life energy starts running to that part.

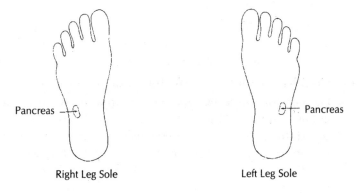

Right Leg Sole   Left Leg Sole

Fig. 4.1 Acupressure area for Pancreas in the Soles

72

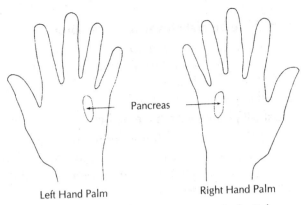

Left Hand Palm   Right Hand Palm

Fig. 4.2 Acupressure area for Pancreas in the Palms

Common Doubts and Their Clarifications Regarding Diabetes

Q. 1   **Is diabetes inherited?**

A.   Yes. If both parents have diabetes, the probability is that their children will develop the disease at some stage in their life. If a diabetic marries a non-diabetic, who has family history of diabetes, there is a chance of their children getting this disease.

Q. 2   **Does infection cause diabetes?**

A.   Not directly as such, but it is known that infection will aggravate or intensify a pre-existing diabetes and make the condition more apparent. Such infections are usually those of skin (boils), respiratory passages (cough and colds) or urinary tract (burning on passing urine).

Q. 3   **Will the eating of an excessive amount of sweets cause diabetes?**

A.   Usually not, but it may aggravate and bring to light an underlying tendency towards the disease.

Q. 4   **How does emotional strain affect diabetes?**

A.   Diabetes may become worse or get out of control by emotional or psychological strain. Sometimes diabetes for first time is brought to light during such a stress.

Q. 5   **Is diabetes infectious?**

A.   No. By mere contact or living with person suffering from diabetes, one cannot get this disease.

Q. 6   **Can there be diabetes without symptoms?**

A.   Yes. Mild case may have no symptoms whatsoever. The disease in such a case may be discovered accidentally by the finding of sugar on routine urine analysis or by blood sugar determination.

Q. 7   **Must all people who have diabetes take insulin?**

A.   No. This depends on the severity and age of onset of the diabetes. Many patients can be controlled adequately by diet alone while some, in addition, by the oral medications.

Q. 8   **Has one to take the special diabetic diet always?**

A.   The principles of diet remain the same. Certain articles have to be avoided. Intake of calories is adjusted depending on the body weight. Those who are overweight must reduce; underweight individuals are given additional calories to make up for their small weight.

Q. 9   **Can a diabetic eat more than his allowance and cover this with increased dosage of oral drugs or insulin?**

A.   No. It will start a vicious circle. The control of diabetes in such patients will become very haphazard. Dietetic restrictions may at no stage be relaxed especially in obese persons.

Q. 10   **Can diabetics keep a fast?**

A.   Overweight diabetics will certainly reduce weight by fasting and it is good for them. Those who are underweight and on large doses of insulin should not do so; or else should reduce the dosage of insulin on such days.

Q. 11   **Can all diabetics derive benefit from the oral medications for control of their diabetes?**

A.   No. Only a few patients will respond to this treatment. Usually they are over forty years in age and have an insulin requirement of less than 40 units per day. A prior test can indicate if a patient will respond to the oral tablets available.

Q. 12   **Can insulin be taken by mouth?**

A.   No, it must be injected under the skin, because if taken orally, it is destroyed in the gut before getting absorbed.

Q. 13 Once a patient has had to take insulin for his diabetes, does it mean that he will have to take it for the rest of his life?

A. Generally speaking, this is so, although there may be exceptions to this rule. This is, however, not like an addiction to opium.

Q. 14 How can a patient tell if his diabetes is being controlled?

A. a. By examination of his own urine for sugar

   b. By having a blood sugar test done at regular intervals

   c. By noting the presence or absence of diabetic symptoms such as excessive thirst, excessive hunger, weight loss, weakness etc.

Q. 15 How often should the urine be tested?

A. Always on rising in the morning and two hours after a main meal. If there is suspicion of the diabetic acidosis or superadded infection, it should be tested more frequently.

Q. 16 Are diabetics particularly prone to infection?

A. Yes, in addition their ability to combat infection is poorer if untreated than that of non-diabetic patient. For this reason, a diabetic must be particularly careful in his personal hygiene and consult his physician as soon as any infection takes place.

Q. 17 Should diabetics have children?

A. If both parents are diabetic, they should realize that their children can have this disease. If they decide to have children, they should know of their responsibility to keep a careful watch for early symptoms of the disease in their offspring whose future may depend on its prompt recognition.

Q. 18 Can diabetic patients be operated upon safely?

A. Yes, With modern methods of management, the diabetic patient can be operated upon with almost as much safety as the non-diabetic patient.

Q. 19 Why a diabetic easily contracts infections?

A.   The glucose rich blood of a diabetic provides optimum conditions for the rapid growth and reproduction of micro-organisms causing infection. A diabetic easily catches infection of skin, gums, and the respiratory tract.

Q. 20 Why there is delayed healing of wound infection in diabetics?

A.   Diabetes affects the small blood vessels and nerves leading to a decrease in blood supply of the skin and derangement of skin sensations. Besides the natural resistance power of the body also decreases in diabetic patient. This is the reason of delayed healing of wound infection.

Q. 21 Why diabetics often complain of pain in legs?

A.   In diabetics, the blood vessels of hands and legs get narrowed resulting in reduced blood supply. This leads to onset of pain in the legs.

Q. 22 Does diabetes lead to increase in blood lipids?

A.   Yes, Insulin has a fat sparing effect. But if insulin is deficient, fats easily get converted into fatty acid to provide energy to the body. Hence triglycerides increase in the blood.

Q. 23 Is high blood pressure quite common in diabetes?

A.   Yes, it is found that 50% diabetics have also high blood pressure.

Q. 24 How diabetes leads to 'Gangrene' of toe or foot?

A.   Gangrene is defined as the death of a part of a tissue or an organ. Gangrene of the toe or foot is 50-60 times more common in diabetics than in healthy persons. Without proper care, even a trivial injury to the toe or the foot may result in gangrene. Narrowing of the blood vessels, poor resistance power and untoward changes of the nervous system are said to be responsible for such proneness of diabetics to gangrene. Gangrene usually necessitates amputation of the affected part to keep the patient alive.

Q. 25 **Why is there excess and frequent urination in diabetics?**

A. The sugar escaping through the kidneys, carries alongwith it a lot of water. A diabetic, therefore passes a lot of urine.

Q. 26 **Why is dryness of mouth and excessive thirst found in diabetics?**

A. This symptom is the result of efforts by the body to compensate for the fluids lost through excessive urine.

Q. 27 **Why is excessive hunger present in diabetics?**

A. In diabetes, glucose can't enter the various body cells. Thus the cells starve inspite of being bathed by glucose rich serum. This cellular starvation leads to excessive hunger.

Q. 28 **Why do diabetics suffer loss of weight?**

A. When the cells can't utilize glucose, the body disintegrates stored fats to provide the cells with necessary energy. Hence the person loses weight.

Q. 29 **Why is weakness and fatigue felt by diabetic?**

A. In diabetes, body also disintegrates stored muscle protein to nourish the starving cells. This is the cause of undue weakness and fatigue.

Q. 30 **Why a diabetic shows mental confusion, forgetfulness, disorientation, lack of concentration and mental fatigue?**

A. Diabetic shows these symptoms because brain cells also are not able to utilize the available glucose and remains undernourished.

Q. 31 **Why a diabetic feels sexual debility?**

A. General weakness, disintegration of muscle protein, mental depression and undesirable changes in blood circulatory and nervous system give rise to this problem.

Q. 32 **Why is numbness of limbs and changes in skin sensations felt by diabetic?**

A. Since nervous system of a diabetic is affected due to not being properly nourished by glucose, hence these symptoms arise.

5. Cervical Spondylosis

Cervical Spondylosis is the *degeneration (or wear and tear) of the spinal discs in the cervical spine.* Cervical spine is made up of seven vertebrae. They are joined to each other by intervertebral discs and ligaments. It is curved with convexity forward. The maximum point of convexity is at the level of disc between the 5th and 6th vertebra. The spondylosis is most common in this disc because this point is the point of maximum stress.

In the process of degeneration, disc loses its water and becomes dry. A disc in its healthy state is soft and elastic though strong. Since it is made of elastic fibres it can be compressed and compression of several discs in harmony can produce a smooth bend in the spine whenever so desired.

However when disc becomes degenerated, its elastic fibers no longer exhibit the elasticity, they become hard and break under stress. The intervertebral disc gets worn out and thinned. Due to this, the edges of the vertebral bodies start rubbing against each other

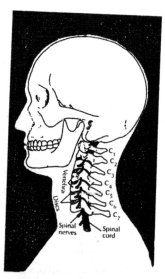

Fig. 5.1 Anatomy of Cervical Spine

and develop *bony spikes called spurs or osteophytes.* They are pointed and sharp. They can be seen on the X-rays. If one of these pointed spurs pokes into the nerve root, it causes severe pain in the arm. They can also cause compression of the spinal cord and can produce paralysis in the hands. A degenerated disc can also bulge out of its normal position commonly known as 'Slipped Disc' in which case it can compress a nerve root causing pain. Slipped disc can also occur due to an accident, sudden fall or blow on the neck. (To know more details about anatomy of disc, disc degeneration, disc prolapse, please refer chapter 13). Movement of the degenerated spine is not smooth as the elasticity of the discs is lost.

Spondylosis occurs normally in the four lower vertebrae i. e. 4th to 7th. It rarely occurs in the upper three vertebrae mainly because they are not subject to much stress. Pain of cervical spondylosis is always felt behind the neck and is never felt in front of neck. When the pain due to Cervical Spondylosis is intense, it can travel down the shoulders and back of the arm upto the elbow joint and sometimes upto hands and fingers. Depending upon which nerve root is affected, the pain will be felt in the corresponding finger.

It is important to understand that the pain of coronary heart disease or angina goes along the inner side of the arm and travels more frequently upto the fingers. Moreover the movement of neck doesn't aggravate the heart pain. But in case of Cervical Spondylosis the pain becomes more by movement of neck. Further heart pain is usually felt on the left side.

Normally degeneration of the discs is an age related phenomena. If an X-ray of the spine is done at the age of 40 years, 30% of them will show degenerative changes and at the age of 50, almost 50% will show evidence of Cervical Spondylosis. At the age of 70, all the vertebrae may show spondylotic changes reducing the flexibility of spinal movement but it is not necessary that they will cause pain because nerve root may not have been affected by them.

When a nerve root is affected in Cervical Spondylosis, it can produce the following symptoms

1. Pain
2. Numbness
3. Stiffness

If a disc slips into the canal and compresses the whole spinal cord, sometimes the paralysis of hands can occur. The compression of the cord can also occur by bony spurs as mentioned earlier.

Treatment

In case of intense pain in the neck due to Cervical Spondylosis associated with or without weakness in the arm, usually the following steps may be followed:

1. **Stoppage of Neck Movement:** All activities which cause movement of the neck must be immediately halted. There is a lot of vibrations and jerks in the neck during travelling and it is advisable to stop travelling and stay away from the office for a few days.

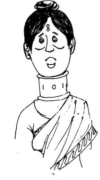

A Cervical Collar (see Fig. 5.2) is advisable to restrict undue movements of the neck. For first few days it is advisable to use collar even while sleeping to avoid

Fig. 5.2

inadvertent twisting of neck in sleep. During sleep, the neck should be in 10 to 15° flexed position rather than neutral or extended position. A normal size pillow causes excessive flexion. This should be avoided. One easy way to support the weak cervical spine while lying is to use Cervical Pillow as shown in following figure.

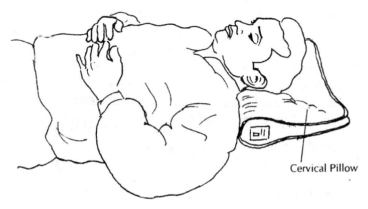

Cervical Pillow

Fig. 5.3

2. **Pain Killers:** Analgesic is advised to get immediate relief from pain. Very rarely it is necessary to take injectable analgesics. Unless the severe pain is reduced by analgesics, no other preventive or long term measures to treat the disease can be initiated.

3. **Heat Treatment:** Whenever there is pain in the joints, the muscles encircling that joint become tight and reduce the mobility of the joint as a protective mechanism. In fact what nature tries to do through muscle spasm we try to do by wearing a Cervical Collar. When the tension in the muscles becomes too much, they generate pain.

   Heat is the best agent to relax the muscles. Many home remedies can be used in this context e.g. hot water bags, electrical heating pads, infrared lamps. One easy way to provide heat to the aching neck is while taking hot shower bath. Allow shower hot water to fall on the back of your neck.

   The more preferable treatments are Short Wave Diathermy and Ultrasound Heat if they are practically possible by visiting a physiotherapist as they provide deep penetrating heat.

4. **Traction:** Traction is quite effective when a slipped disc presses a nerve root. Traction increases the intervertebral disc space and therefore the pressure of disc on the nerve root is released. Method of giving traction to neck is shown in the (Fig. 5.4). Traction can be intermittent or steady traction kept up for some time. If traction fails to reduce pain in 24 to 48 hours, there is little reason to insist on its use any further.

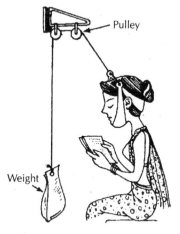

Fig. 5.4

Stretching of the neck can also be done manually as shown in the following figure.

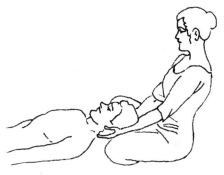

Fig. 5.5

5. **Massage:** Massage is a very effective way for relaxing the tense muscles of the neck. Various massage techniques have been illustrated in the following figures.

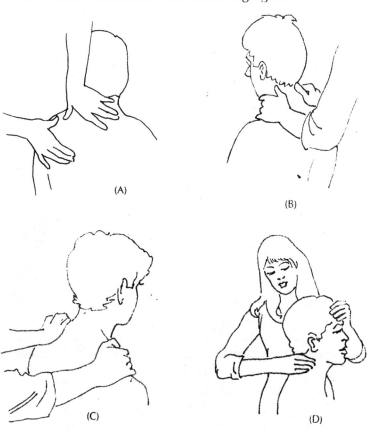

(A)

(B)

(C)

(D)

Fig. 5.6

You can also do self-massage by various techniques illustrated below.

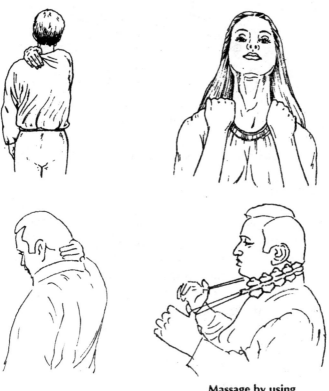

Fig. 5.6A

Massage by using acupressure roller

6. **Acupressure:** Acupressure on both sides of spine on the upper back is found very relaxing and soothing for the sufferers of pain of Cervical Spondylosis. This acupressure can be given while the patient is sitting or lying in prone position as shown in Fig. 5.7.

This acupressure can be given by spine roller also as shown in Fig. 5.7 A.

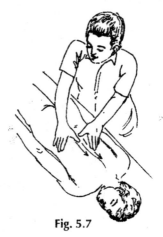

Fig. 5.7

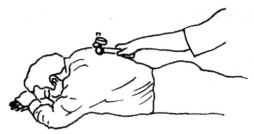

Fig. 5.7A

7. **Strengthening Neck Muscles:** As already explained spine is more vulnerable to injury when the muscles associated with it are weak. If the muscles associated with spine are strong, the extra load can be shared by the muscles if the spine is weak. Various exercises to strengthen the muscles of neck, shoulders and upper back are shown in the following figures.

However these exercises should be taken up only when the initial intense pain is subsided by the conservative treatments described before.

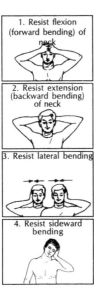

Fig. 5.8

8. **Exercises for Loosening Stiff Muscles:** After the initial pain has subsided, you can start exercises for loosening stiff neck, upper back and shoulder muscles as shown in Fig. 5.9.

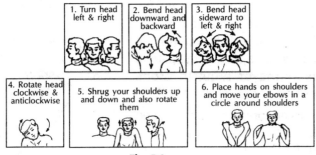

Fig. 5.9

A Few Words about the Surgery

This question is most often asked when a patient should go for surgery in case he is suffering from Cervical Spondylosis.

If a patient has severe pain or significant weakness or paresis or increasing numbness and sensory loss, then surgery is advisable. Similarly if a patient doesn't respond conservative treatment (as described before) for the required number of days, then surgical intervention should be considered. Sometimes pain might get diminished but paresis and numbness remain or get worse. In this case surgery should be considered. Continued numbness suggests that nerve root is being held compressed to such an extent that its function may soon be lost.

The purpose of operation is to remove all the pressure on the nerve root and the spinal cord, provide more room for both nerve roots and the spinal cord and stabilize the unstable vertebrae by doing a fusion of the two vertebrae by interposing a piece of bone graft in between when necessary. There are a variety of operative procedures. Some are done from behind the neck and some by approaching the neck from the front. The intervertebral disc between two vertebrae is removed and the empty space is replaced by a piece of bone cut to the necessary shape and size to fit exactly into the space created. This extra piece of bone known as bone graft is usually obtained from the patients hip bone (iliac bone). If the spine shows abnormal movement or instability, the logic is to fuse the spine at the level of instability.

Whether operation will cure your problem completely or partially depends upon many things. For example if the numbness is due to compression of the nerve root, numbness will definitely improve but if a nerve is damaged, the numbness will persist even after the operation. It is observed that if the patients come for operation at an early stage whenever such types of symptoms as numbness, weakness in arms and/or legs are found, then the better it is. Delay can produce irreversible changes leading to uncertainty of results in operation. Doing the operation too late merely prevents further damage but can't undo the damage already occurred.

It is interesting to note that only a small percentage of patients are required to go in for surgery. Sixty to Seventy percent of the patients carry on well with conservative treatments.

6. Slip Disc and Sciatica

Before going into detailed discussion of the Slip-disc treatment and Sciatica first we should properly understand the anatomy of disc and vertebra.

Anatomy of Spinal Discs

Discs are cushions of cartilage that separate any two vertebrae. They are very tough yet flexible structures. They act as shock absorbers getting compressed when weight is put upon the spine and springing back to their original shape when the weight is taken away. Disc dampens the force which comes from your feet when you walk or run so that it doesn't go to the brain to cause damage. Discs all together constitute about one third of the total length of the spine. It is because of these elastic discs that you are able to bend your spine in many directions (flexion, extension, rotation, lateral bending).

The disc absorbs water, becomes taut and packs the joint to act as a wedge between the vertebrae. When discs are fully hydrated with water and firm, they are effective wedges, particularly in the lumbar region reducing the demand on the back muscles. If the discs are not fully hydrated and their wedge quality is poor it becomes the increasing responsibility of the back muscles to keep the body upright.

During the day when you are upright and moving, the force of your weight in motion (which is more than your static weight) will force water out of your discs of the person into the vertebrae above and below. This release can cause a shrinkage in height of the person of about one and half to two centimetres during 12 hours. During the night, while you sleep, the discs absorb water from its surroundings. Disc has no blood vessels and nerves of its own. There must be enough free water in the region for it to be able to rehydrate itself. Hence the importance of more water intake for those who have a tendency of low back pain. Bed rest recommended in treatment of disc problems prevents shrinkage of discs and allows full rehydration of the discs. Incidentally in the case of astronauts travelling in space, the discs swell considerably due to weightlessness in space and the height of astronauts increase as much as two inches.

The disc is composed of an outer fibrous material called 'Annulus fibrosus' and an inner pulpy substance called 'Nucleus pulposus' . It is the property and function of the pulpy substance of the disc to absorb or give up its water. The fibrous part firmly fixes the disc to bony edges of the vertebrae.

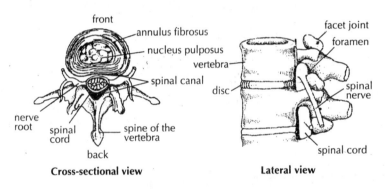

Fig. 6.1 Anatomy of Disc and Vertebra

Degeneration of Spinal Discs

With the advancement of age, thinning and degeneration of discs including general wear and tear of spine takes place and it starts in everybody from the age of 25 to 30 years. By the age of 60 years it is quite advanced. With the degeneration of the disc its load bearing capacity decreases and spinal movement at that level is restricted. When disc is completely degenerated it is like lifeless mass and can't be regenerated. Slip disc is invariably associated with degeneration of the disc because with degenerated or weakened disc it is easier for **'Nucleus pulposus'** to tear through **'Annulus fibrosus'** (outer part of the disc) and bulge outwards.

With the degeneration of disc, there are other implications as well. For example there is formation of **'osteophytes'** (bony spurs at the edge of vertebrae). This further restricts the movement of the spine at that level. The facet joints in the back of spine must be maintained at a delicate non-weight bearing relationship for their movement regulating

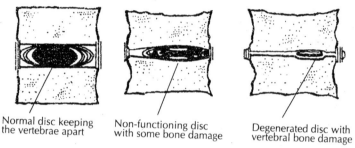

| Normal disc keeping the vertebrae apart | Non-functioning disc with some bone damage | Degenerated disc with vertebral bone damage |

Fig. 6.2 Thinning and degeneration of disc

responsibilities. A well hydrated disc brings this about by effectively packing the joint, whereas a thin disc will force these facet joints to become weight bearing becoming in the long run a cause for arthritis. Similarly the space for exit of nerve root (also called foramen) is also reduced with the thinning of discs and jamming of facet joints.

Pressure Changes on Spinal Discs

The figure shown below (Fig. 6.3) shows the percentage change in load acting on the lower lumbar discs with various positions of the body. The standing position is taken as the reference point and is set to zero. Taking the upright standing intradiscal pressure as the norm, it should be noted that a five-degree tilt will increase the pressure by 25%, unsupported sitting will increase it by 50%, and lying supine decreases the pressure by 50%. By marked forward flexion and rotation, the intradiscal pressure may increase by as much as 400%. For these reasons, one can see how it is best to lift weights with a straight spine and bent knees instead of by forward bending of spine so as to avoid excess pressure on the spine.

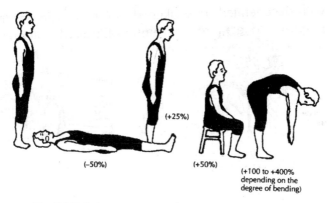

Fig. 6.3 Relative pressure on disc in various positions w.r.t. standing position

Loads most damaging to disc tissue are bending and torsional loads, especially if applied suddenly. It is observed in experiments that if spine is subjected to very high compressive load applied gradually, there is no injury to the fibers of annulus (outer part of disc) and failure of the annular fibers occur when subjected to bending and torsional loads. It has been noticed that in case of healthy disc, even a compressive load enough to damage the body of vertebra is not sufficient to damage the disc. But of course, when the disc becomes weak and degenerated, the condition becomes different and in that case the person should avoid the axial compressive loads also on the spine.

Mechanism of Slip-Disc

The otherwise tough annulus fibrosus (outer part of disc) is somewhat weak at the back and the sides of the disc. If it gives way or gets torn, it may allow the nucleus pulposus to bulge out. If this bulge presses against one of the spinal nerves, the result is pain. Infact the disc doesn't slip, it only bulges. This phenomena, in medical parlance is also termed as **Disc protrusion/Disc prolapse/Disc herniation** etc. This condition normally results when there is too much pressure or lateral strain on the spine. It is usually the result of some sudden violent episodes such as a fall, an accident, sudden twisting of spine, suddenly lifting a heavy object, sudden forward bending of spine associated with lifting an object. The slip disc mostly

89

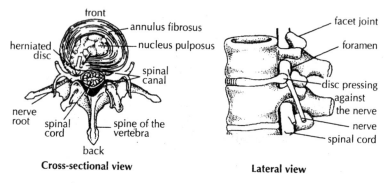

Cross-sectional view   Lateral view

Fig. 6.4 Nerve pinching by slipped disc

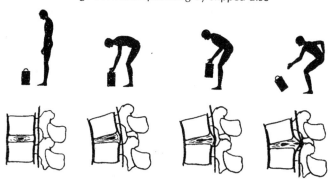

Fig. 6.5 Disc protrusion during forward bending in case of weak disc

occurs at the level of L-5 & S-1 (i.e. between 5th lumbar vertebra and 1st sacral vertebra) because this disc receives the maximum pressure and this is the point where the spine transfers the load of the upper part of body to the hip bones and thence to legs. But disc can slip at L2-L3 and L3-L4 level also.

Symptoms and Diagnosis of Slip-Disc

In addition to the pain in the lower back, the patient of slip disc also complains of pain radiating or shooting down into the back of leg (along the course of sciatic nerve which gets irritated by the pressure of disc on this nerve). During the physical examination, the patient may not be able to raise the leg without pain (called the Straight leg raising test). Then there may be neurological changes in sensations of the legs e.g. feeling of numbness, tingling etc. There may be changes in the reflexes of knee and ankle. Then there may be difference of sensations in both the legs.

One more simple and frequently used diagnostic method is to see if the fingertip pressure between the bony posterior processes of the spine or their sides produces a local pain. This is a good indication that the disc has produced soft tissue pressure on the nerve or the spinal cord which is further aggravated by pressing of the tissue above the aggravated area by the finger.

X-ray is not sufficient diagnosis for a herniated disc. It may at best give the indication of degeneration and thinning of discs. When patient complains continuous pain in the leg and there is an increasing loss of nerve function, then a more sophisticated test known as M.R.I. (Magnetic Resonance Imaging) should be got done which gives the accurate picture of the area.

Treatment of Slip Disc by Exercises

Although in the complicated cases and chronic pain, surgery is the only answer where the protruding disc is removed by surgery, but in less complicated cases the exercises mentioned below can be useful. However these exercises should be done only when the original pain is subsided by bed rest, analgesics or pain killers and other simple measures (e.g. heat treatment through hot water bag/heating pad/hot packs or fomentation). Another precaution to be taken in exercises is that they should be done slowly without any jerks. If you find any increasing discomfort or pain by doing any exercises, discontinue that exercise. Use your intuition in this regard.

Further forward bending should be avoided by a Slip-disc patient. If at all forward bending is to be done (either in routine movement or during some exercises), it should be done with knees bent. With knees bent, bending mostly takes place at hip joint and lower back is relieved from the stress. Similarly if during forward bending spine is supported by hands placed on the ground, then also there is minimal stress on lower back (see Fig.6.15) because in this case body weight is being supported by the four limbs directly and not by spine. From yoga point of view there are mainly the following approaches which can help in alleviating the pain of Slipped-disc and Sciatica.

1. Good Postures: One should always maintain good postures. Good postures are formulated on the principle that the natural curve of the spine is maintained i.e. it is not distorted or exaggerated in any posture and your pelvis remains balanced. Further body is kept in symmetrical position with respect to central axis while standing, sitting and walking. Load bearing is also done in such a manner that it is symmetrically lifted and there is minimum eccentricity. In this condition there is minimum strain on the back.

Some of the good postures are shown below in the form of Do's and Dont's.

Do's	Pictures
1. Always use firm mattress.	
2. Ideal lying position is side lying with hips and knees slightly bent.	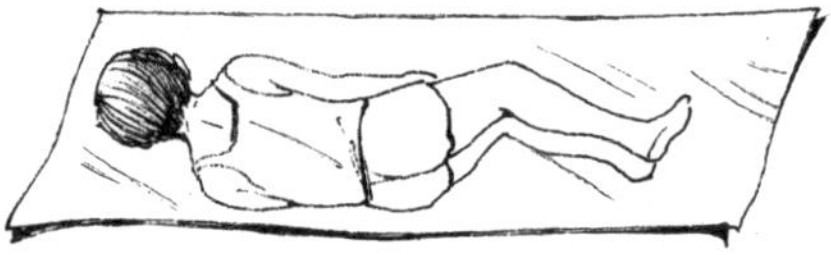
3. If you lie in back lying position keep hips and knees bent. A pillow can be kept under the knees otherwise.	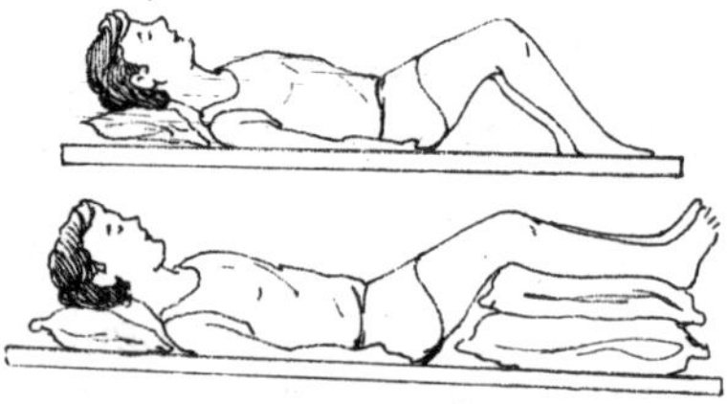
4. How to sit up from lying position. (a) bend both hips and knees. (b) Come to side lying bearing body weight on both arms.	(a) (b)

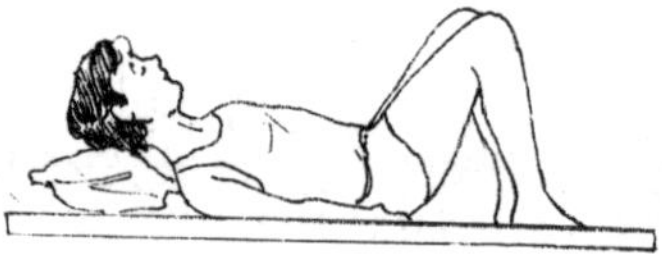

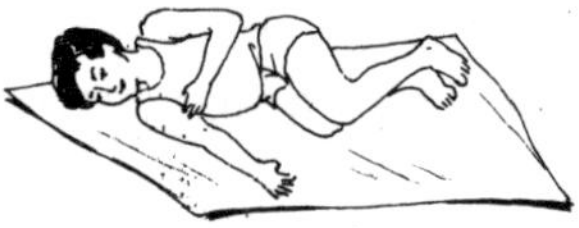

Fig. 6.6 (Contd.....)

Do's	Pictures
(c) Come up, with both legs coming down simultaneously.	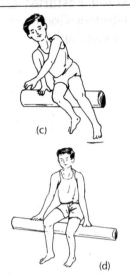 (c)
(d) While sitting, take support of both arms.	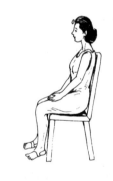 (d)
5. Sit erect on a chair with back support keeping your back against the support.	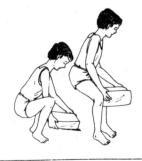
6. To lift objects from the ground, first squat with back straight, hold the object, and get up slowly straightening your knees.	

Dont's	Pictures
1. Avoid mattress that are sagging.	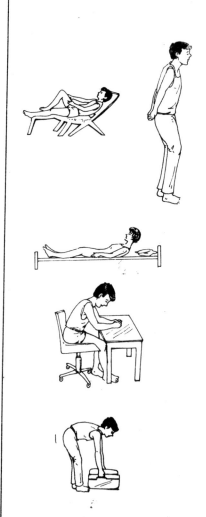
2. Avoid slouching while standing or sitting.	
3. Avoid sitting up straight form back lying positions.	
4. Avoid sitting away from the working table, Sit at a closest possible distance.	
5. Don't bend while lifting objects from the ground.	
6. Avoid lifting heavy weight (above 10 to 15 kg.)	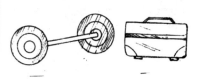

Fig. 6.6 Do's and Dont's for maintaining good postures

2. Relaxing Back Muscles: With pain in the back, muscles around that region invariably remain tight and muscles when remained continuously tight and contracted, themselves start paining. Hence it is desirable to relax these muscles frequently by stretching exercises. Some of the back muscles loosening exercises are shown below:

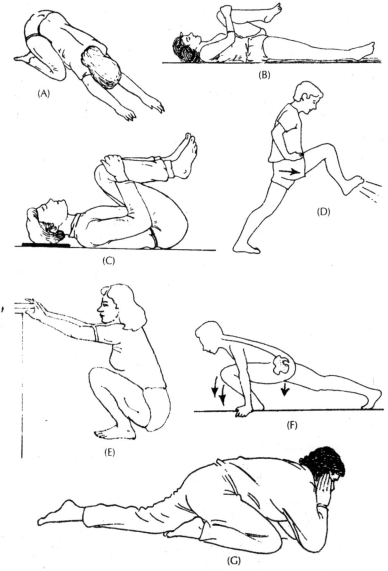

Fig. 6.7

3. Loosening Hip Joint: Loosening of hip joint is essential to ease pressure on the lower back because if hip joint is tight, there is more pressure on the back while bending and this will worsen your Slip disc problem. Although many of the back muscles relaxing exercise loosen hip joint also but some additional exercises are also shown below:

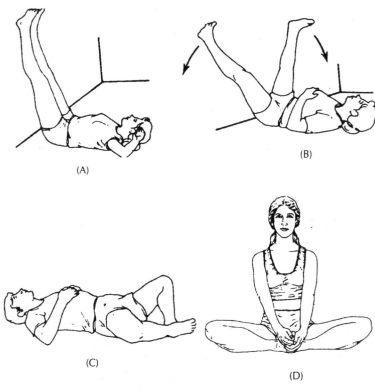

(A)

(B)

(C)

(D)

Fig. 6.8

4. Strengthening Back Muscles: When back muscles are weak, they can't support the spine well and can't keep the spine and pelvis in a balanced position. When the muscles of the back are strong, they can also easily relieve the disc of bearing excess load and can share extra load. Further strong muscles also help in realigning the spinal vertebrae in their proper axis. Some of the exercises for strengthening back muscles are shown below:

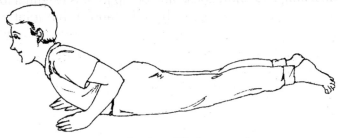

(A) Cobra Pose (Bhujangasana)

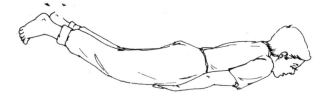

(B) Locust Pose (Shalabhasana)

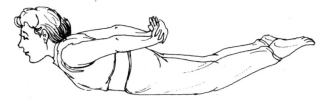

(C) Naukasana-Combined exercise to strengthen upper back and lower back muscles and improve alignment of low back, chest and neck vertebrae

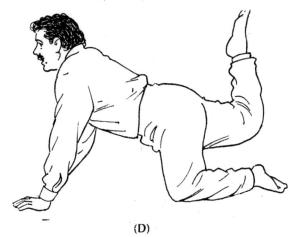

(D)

Fig. 6.9

5. **Strengthening of Abdominal Muscles:** Strengthening of abdominal muscles is equally important because abdominal muscles support the front of the spine. With weak abdominal muscles. Abdomen will sag forward leading to forward tilting of pelvis which distorts the natural curve of spine and makes pelvis unbalanced making spine more vulnerable to injury.

There is a mechanism called 'Hydraulic Sac Mechanism' which is created by coordinated contraction of stomach muscles, back muscles, the diaphragm and pelvic floor muscles. When these muscles tighten simultaneously, the abdominal cavity which is an enclosed sac of fluid gives added support to the spine so that when the spine is called on to lift a heavy load, the total weight is not transmitted entirely through the spine. Some of the exercises for strengthening abdominal muscles are shown below:

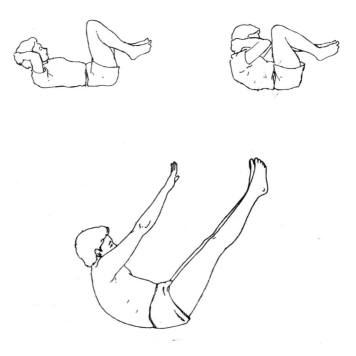

Fig. 6.10

6. Spinal Extension Exercises: They are the key exercises in the treatment of Slip-disc. Spinal extension exercises help to retract the disc back to its normal position. In the spinal extension exercises (Backward bending) the ligaments attached to the front of the disc are stretched when the front angle is opened up. In this process they (ligaments) draw the disc back into its intervertebral space and away from the nerve root or the spinal cord. At the same time, by creating a space in the position where the disc used to be, a force of vacuum will be generated which sucks water for rehydration of discs and cartilage (covering the bony vertebra) enhancing its lubrication and gliding property.

Since these exercises are the very foundation for Slip Disc treatment, they are being explained in detail below:

Exercise 1

Take two big round pillows (or otherwise you can take two normal pillows in place of one big round pillow). Place them on the ground about one and a half feet apart. Kneel on the pillows such that your knees rest on the rear pillows and your chest rests on front pillows and hands comfortably resting on the ground ahead comfortably with elbows bent as shown in Fig. 6.11. This will position your abdomen and the painful area of the back in the hollow between the pillows. Your body should be off the ground by 5 to 6" when you lie on the pillows.

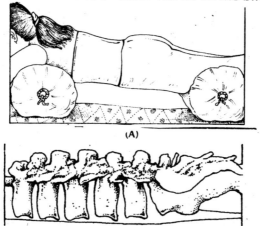

(A)

(B) Position of spine representing the posture in (A)

Fig. 6.11 *(Contd....)*

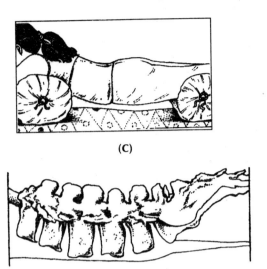

(C)

(D) Position of spine representing the posture shown in **(C)**

Fig. 6.11

Now all that is involved is rhythmic movement of spine up and down in the hollow. When you go down, it opens up the front angle of disc spaces as shown in Fig. 6.11 which helps to pull the disc to its normal location.

Exercise 2

Lie on your back. Bend your feet and bring them as close to your buttocks as possible. Keeping this position, raise your buttocks off the ground as high as possible. Remain in this position for as long as you can comfortably stay. Then come down slowly, repeat it a few times.

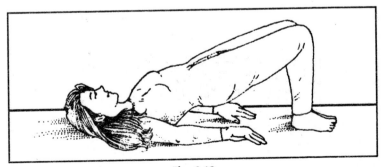

Fig. 6.12

Exercise 3

Lie on your stomach with palms of hands placed near respective shoulder. Straighten arms while inhaling. Throw chest out as far as possible. Curve backwards to its and look at the ceiling, stretching neck backwards fullest extent. In this position practically the whole weight of the body is carried by the arms.

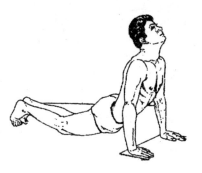

Fig. 6.13

Now reverse your body curvature. Your body should form an inverted V. Your feet should remain flat on the ground. You will feel a good stretch behind your ankle and knee in this position.

Do these two positions in a rhythmic movement, few times. Finally come down kneeling on your knees as shown in Fig. 6.15. Then slide back with the support of your hands into position of Vajrasana and then stand up. Never stand up directly from the exercise posture to avoid strain on your back.

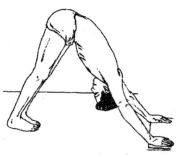

Fig. 6.14

Exercise 4

Sit in the position of Vajrasana. Inhale and then while exhaling stretch your hands ahead and bend your body forward from the buttocks. You can put your head on the floor if you feel so. Buttocks shouldn't preferably be raised above the heels while bending. See Fig. 6.7A in this chapter.

Now come forward gradually while keeping your hand in the same position on the ground and moving hips forward (see Fig. 6.15). Inhale and bend back keeping legs and feet together. Look up and back, keeping your hips lowered.

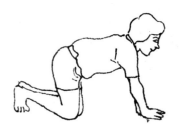

Fig. 6.15 Intermediate position   **Fig. 6.16** Final position

Now go back to the previous position (Fig. 6.7A) and do this exercise a few times.

Exercise 5

Stand erect with feet 6″ apart and parallel. Inhale and stretch your arms up and arch back from the waist pushing the hips forward and keeping legs straight. Keep your hips tightened which helps in giving firm support to the lower back, neck and head should hang back loosely looking at the ceiling.

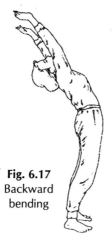

Fig. 6.17 Backward bending

Exercise 6

This exercise is nothing but what is called 'Dhanurasana' in Yoga. Lie down on your front, head down. Inhale and bend your knees up and clasp your ankles with your hands. Inhaling raise your head and chest up and simultaneously pull you ankles up, lifting the knees and thighs off the floor. Arch backward and look up. Then exhale and come back slowly to normal position.

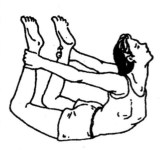

Fig. 6.18

Those who can do 'chakrasana' may also find it useful. But it should be done slowly without jerk. It is difficult for most of the people and hence is being omitted here. 'Bhujangasana' and 'Shalbhasana' shown in Fig. 6.9 are also very good for Slip-disc patients.

7. Miscellaneous Exercises: Following exercises have also been found useful in relieving the disc pressure on the nerve.

Exercise 1

Lie down on stomach. Lift one leg and slowly bend it with the help of hand of that side so that the heel touches the buttock. Then follow the same process with the other leg. Then take both the legs together and bend them slowly on both the buttocks simultaneously. Remain in this position for a few minutes. If you prefer you can also raise your head and chest up in this position.

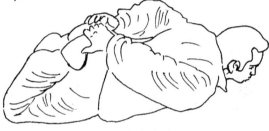

Fig. 6.19

Exercise 2

Lie on your back. Bend one leg and put the foot on the thigh of another leg. Now move the knee of the bent leg up and down. Do the same with the other leg.

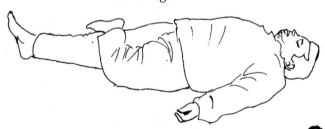

Fig. 6.20

This exercise can also be done while sitting on chair as shown.

Exercise shown in Fig. 6.8 C in this chapter is also useful in this regard.

Fig. 6.21

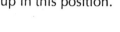

Exercise 3 ·

Lie on a slant board with your feet elevated and anchored in the strap at the end of the board. Take your hands over your head. (See Fig. 2.6 in this book). In this position, your whole body including the spine is stretched with the help of gravity. It is a kind of natural traction for the spine which increases the intervertebral space and pulls the disc back freeing the nerve of its pressure. By this stretch, the spine also gets correctly aligned and any defect in its curvature tends to get rectified.

Exercise 4

Try dorsi flexion of your ankle joints keeping your leg straight. It stretches your entire back of leg. It can better be done by somebody else as shown in Fig 6.22. It helps reducing the pain of Sciatica.

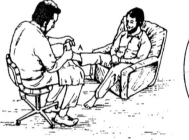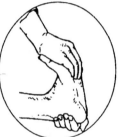

Enlarged view at 'A'

Fig. 6.22

Exercise shown below in Fig. 6.23 also stretches the back of leg effectively and reduces the pain of Sciatica. In this exercise, you walk around the room keeping the knees and elbows straight and ensuring that feet lie flat on the floor. However for doing this exercise, first you should kneel on the knee with your hands on the ground (see Fig. 6.23) and then come to this pose so that no load comes on the lumbar spine. Similarly while coming back to your original posture, reverse the above sequence and never stand up suddenly.

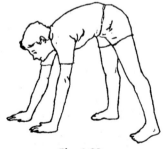

Fig. 6.23

Exercise 5 (Pelvic Tilt Exercise)

When the pelvis is tipped forward, it creates an unnatural strain on the spine and makes it weak and vulnerable to injury.

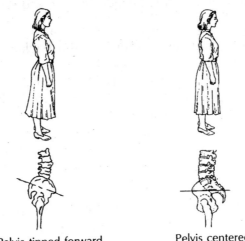

Pelvis tipped forward   Pelvis centered
creating hollow in the back

Fig. 6.24

Pelvic tilt exercise as shown in the following figure should be done to correct the problem of hyperlordosis (excessive hollow in the back) and to bring pelvis in central balanced position which is a position of least strain and maximum stability of the spine. In this exercise we flatten the hollow of the back by contracting and tightening the stomach muscles.

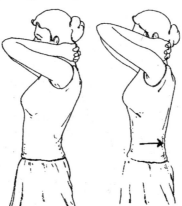

Fig. 6.25

105

Miscellaneous Home Remedies

Following miscellaneous treatments have also been found useful for alleviating the pain of slip-disc and sciatica.

1. **Massage on the Back of Legs:** Massaging the back of legs is very effective in reducing the backache since the acupuncture meridian B1 which passes through lower back also continues in the back of leg. For massaging the back of leg, ask your patient to lie in prone position. Then work slowly up the leg starting from the ankle and right upto the hips. Use your thumbs or heels of your hands to press gradually up the muscles and flesh of calf, thigh and hips. Let your movement be continuous and rhythmic.

   Now a days hand rollers are also available which you can roll on the back of legs by applying little pressure.

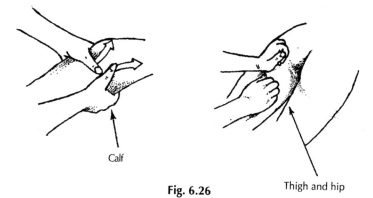

Calf

Fig. 6.26

Thigh and hip

There are two important acupuncture points on this meridian B1 (one at the back of knee and one in the middle of crease below the buttock) as shown in the following figure. Giving intermittent pressure on these points gives substantial relief to backache.

Pressing back of heel and achilli tendon as shown in Fig. 7.12 (Chapter 7) of this book is said to be quite helpful in reducing the pain of sciatica.

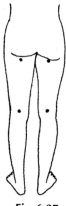

Fig. 6.27

2. **Treating Spinal Reflex on the Foot:** There is an extraordinary similarity between the shape of the spine and the shape of its reflex on the inside of the foot as shown in Fig 6.28. Both have 26 bones and the four arches of the feet mirror the four curves of the spine. According to principles of 'Reflexology' if you work on the reflexes of the foot corresponding to various body parts, that body part starts healing because of the link of the reflex with that part through energy channel (or meridian). Hence if you work on the spinal reflexes on the foot, you are giving

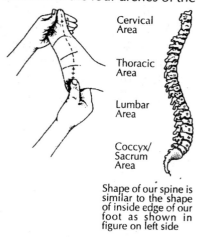

Cervical Area

Thoracic Area

Lumbar Area

Coccyx/ Sacrum Area

Shape of our spine is similar to the shape of inside edge of our foot as shown in figure on left side

Fig. 6.28

healing to your spine also. Now to work on the spinal reflexes, you start pressing at the inside edge of the heel and walk your thumb up gradually towards the big toe along the dotted line shown in the figure. For slip disc patient, the area of the spinal reflex in the foot corresponding to the lumbar curve should be given more massage. Similar reflexes also exist in the hands.

3. **Reiki Treatment:** Give Reiki to your lower back (location of Back Hara chakra) and tip of the spine at the back (Mooladhara chakra) by putting your hands as shown. Reiki

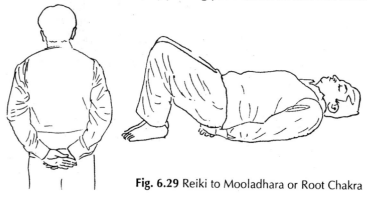

Fig. 6.29 Reiki to Mooladhara or Root Chakra

107

at these points is more easily given in lying position. By giving Reiki here by hands, these portions are stimulated by life energy. Reiki to Mooladhra chakra is specially useful since this chakra controls the full musculoskeletal system of the body and makes it sturdy. While giving Reiki, focus your mind also to that location, this will accelerate the healing. (For more details on how 'Reiki' works, please refer my book **'Healing through Reiki'** from the same publisher).

4. **Heat Treatment:** Heat relieves muscle spasm and brings about dilation of blood vessels thereby improving the blood supply to the affected part and consequent removal of waste products accumulated in muscles.

   Heat can be given to the painful portion by a hot water bag or electrical or heating pad or by a towel soaked in hot water.

   I find the following two ways most convenient for giving heat to the sore back.

   a. Lie down on your back and put hot water rubber bottle below your sacral spine. In this position heat will be going to your lumbo sacral spine while you are just lying relaxed. Moreover keeping the bottle below your sacral part of spine also causes pelvic tilt which is useful for you.

   b. Lie down in a hot water tub as shown is Fig. 6.30 you can also mix some salt in the water for more effectiveness.

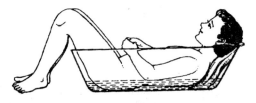

Fig. 6.30

5. **Massage on the Lower Back and Hips:** You can give massage to lower back in various ways to reduce pain. For example:

a. You can apply some pain removing oil or cream (e.g. Seasame oil, Rheumatil oil/gel of 'Dabur') on your lower back and then massage the lower back by the fingers of your hand in a clockwise circular motion.

b. You can give pointed pressure with your thumbs on both sides of spine as shown in Fig. 6.31.

c. You can run a hand roller along the spine starting from the base of spine, upto the upper back by applying a little pressure. (Fig. 6.31A)

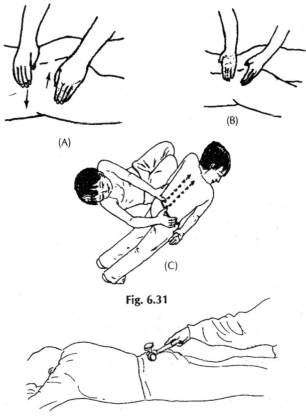

(A)

(B)

(C)

Fig. 6.31

Fig. 6.31A

There is another kind of acupressure roller also by which massage can be given to lower back as shown in the following figure.

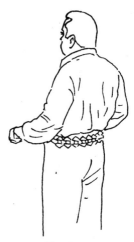

Fig. 6.31B

Note: Acupressure rollers are available in market from nature cure shops or with acpuncturists.

Massage on hips is also very effective for reducing lower backache. It can either be a simple rubbing or stroking massage as shown in Fig. 6.32 or hacking massage as shown in Fig. 6.33 which is more effective. Hacking massage is given by bouncing on the hips with the sides of your hands with hands moving alternately up and down with palms of both hands facing one another.

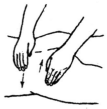

Fig. 6.32

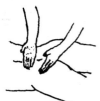

Fig. 6.33

6. Wearing silver ring on the toes (specially on middle toe) or your feet is said to alleviate sciatica pain.

Useful Precautions for Slip-Disc Patient

Once the pain has subsided by taking various measures mentioned in this chapter the following precautions should be routinely taken by a slip disc patient:

1. All sports involving sudden uncontrolled movements should be avoided.

2. Any exercises which overload the back (such as aerobics) should be avoided. Swimming (especially on the back) and walking are, on the other hand, recommended.

3. Forward bending should usually be avoided except with the precaution as mentioned elsewhere in this chapter.

4. All sporting activity must be preceded by a "warm-up".

5. Heavy weight-bearing must be avoided.

6. "Good Postures" should invariably be maintained by a slip-disc patient to prevent undue stress on his back.

7. Asymmetrical body movements, sudden/jerky body movement and lifting of unbalanced loads w.r.t body axis should be avoided.

8. A slip disc patient should always sleep on hard bed. A thin mattress can be used over board or ply but thick sagging mattress should never be used. If a thick mattress is to be used, then 'Ortho mattress' should be used which is specially designed for back patients.

9. Whenever you are on a journey where impacts and jerks are likely to be there (for example, on a rough road), always use lumbar belts (see details ahead).

10. Avoid climbing on steep stairs and ladders as far as possible.

11. If you sit on a chair or sofa where your lower back is not in contact with the back of seat properly, use cushion or lumbar support (see Fig. 6.34).

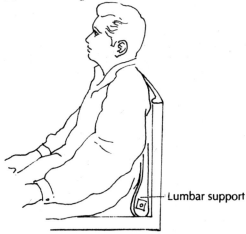

Lumbar support

Fig. 6.34 Sitting with lumbar support

111

Lumbar Belt

Lumbar belt substitutes the action of your muscles. So if your back and abdominal muscles are weak, then belt can compensate for them and provide the necessary support to your spine. But one shouldn't become totally dependent on it because it will tend to further weaken your muscles. It should be used as a temporary measure only.

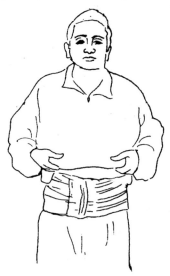

Fig. 6.35 Lumbar Belt

One should continue to strengthen his muscles by suitable exercises and strive to leave dependency on the belt at a certain point of time. When your muscles become strong they become your natural belt to support the spine.

7. Arthritis

What is Arthritis

Arthritis literally refers to 'Pain and inflammation of the joints'. Inflammation is a classical feature of Arthritis. Also it is a defensive mechanism by which the body reacts protectively against an invasion of its tissues. The most often affected joints in arthritis are hips, knees, ankles, elbows and fingers.

Clinical Characteristics of Inflammation

1. Redness
2. Pain
3. Heat
4. Swelling

A few important other clinical features of arthritis are:

1. Loss of mobility/stiffness
2. Instability
3. Deformity

Physiology of Arthritis

Two bones meet at a joint and are connected in a way that permits each to move in relation to the other. At the end of each bone there is a cap of smooth white cartilage which is a tough tissue, which acts as a cushion when the joint is in use. The cartilage thus prevents bone to bone rubbing and consequent wear and tear.

The liquid that lubricates the cartilage is called the **synovial fluid,** contained within the **synovial membrane.** The delicate synovial membrane is protected by a strong, fibrous layer called the 'capsule'.

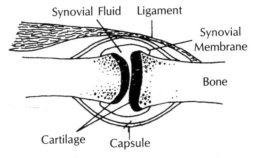

Fig. 7.1 Structure of a Joint

If the circulation of blood and lymphatic fluid in a joint becomes sluggish and the joint fluid (synovial fluid) grows stagnant, the waste products and poisons of cellular metabolism build up in the lubricating fluid (synovial fluid) of the joints rather than being efficiently transported to the skin and kidneys for elimination from the body. Acidic wastes and toxins, accumulated in the joint fluid, irritate the sensitive nerve fibres in the joint causing pain and stiffness. If this situation persists for a long time, the structure of the joint begins to degenerate. The joint fluid begins to dry up, the soft cartilage lining corrodes away and the bones themselves begin to accumulate excessive calcium, forming new bone growth which limits movement. Gradually the whole joint is destroyed and movement becomes impossible.

In a healthy hip, smooth cartilage covers the ends of your hip bones, allowing the ball to glide easily in the socket. Smooth weight-bearing surfaces allow for painless movement.

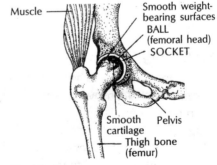

Fig. 7.2 A Healthy Hip Joint

114

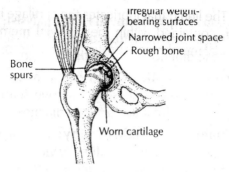

In a problem hip, the cartilage "cushion" wears away, and the bones rub together, becoming rough and pitted. The ball grinds in the socket when you walk, causing pain and stiffness.

Fig. 7.3 A Degenerated Hip Joint

In fact a careful examination and analysis of the synovial fluid can easily provide a clue to determine the type and extent of arthritis.

More specific causes of arthritis will be discussed against the respective type of arthritis.

Laboratory Tests for Diagnosis of Arthritis

1. **ESR (Erythrocyte Sedimentation Rate):** This is a measurement of how fast the RBC collect at the bottom of a glass tube which is filled with a test sample of the blood. *High ESR is found in people with inflammation due to arthritis (and also in some other causes like TB and a few types of cancer).*

2. **Total Blood Count:** It includes RBC count, WBC count, Platelet count, Haemoglobin %, total proteins with Albumin and Globulin levels, c-reactive protein (or CRP) value estimation.

3. **RF Test (or Rheumatoid Factor Test):** It checks if a certain kind of abnormal antibody known as RF is present in the blood. In 70–80% of RA (Rheumatoid Arthritis) cases, RF is present in a quantity higher than 80 I.U.

4. **ANA Test (Anti Nuclear Antibody Test):** This Test is used to determine the presence of another type of abnormal antibody 'Anti DNA' type of ANA.

5. **VDRL Test:** Suggested for patients suffering from syphilis who shows symptoms of arthritis.

6. **Non-Immunological Test:** Tests for estimation of serum enzyme.

7. **Tissue Biopsy (Synovial Fluid Analysis):** In this test, synovial fluid is drawn out from the joint. This test is specially useful in the diagnosis of infective and gouty arthritis.

8. **X-ray, CT, MRI:** X-rays of the affected joints including imaging techniques like isotope scan, CT and MRI can also be helpful to doctor in diagnosis.

9. **Diagnostic Arthroscopy:** It is a procedure using which the doctor can directly view the insides of the joints. The orthopaedic surgeon can do it by inserting an arthroscope, the diameter of which is as small as that of a drinking straw, into the joint through a small hole and move it around to examine the joint tissues such as the cartilage and extent of damage to the joint can be determined.

Types of Arthritis

1. Rheumatoid Arthritis (RA)

2. Osteo arthritis (OA)

3. Infective Arthritis

4. Arthritis associated with Rheumatic Fever

5. Juvenile Chronic Arthritis

6. Gouty Arthritis

7. Psoriatic Arthropathy

8. Ankylosing Spondylitis

Arthritis is also classified as monoarthritis (involving a single joint only) e.g. gouting arthritis and polyarthritis (involving multiple joints) e.g. rheumatoid arthritis.

Rheumatoid Arthritis (RA)

This is a chronic arthritis that typically affects the same joints on the two sides of the body, such as the hands and feet with the symptoms coming and going at different times. RA is one of the more common types of arthritis.

Diagnosis of RA

RA is diagnosed if a patient has at least four of the seven criteria given below:

1. Morning stiffness of the joints for at least one hour for a period of 6 weeks or more

2. Arthritis of three or more joints

3 Arthritis of hand joints

4. Symmetrical arthritis i.e. involving same joints on both sides of the body

5. Presense of RF in the serum of the affected patient

6. Presence of Rheumatoid nodules (observed by a physician)

7. Radiological changes (of the hand and wrist).

The onset of the disease is heralded by symptoms such as fatigue, weight loss, muscle ache (myalgia), early morning stiffness of the joints, arthalgia (joint pain), joint swelling and sometimes fever.

Causes of RA

Many theories have been put forward to find the causes of this disease.

1. **Infection:** The most reasonable theory suggests that RA may be due to some kind of infection by tiny germs called viruses. These are yet unknown. Viruses could find their way into the joints and trigger off inflammation.

2. **Auto Immune Response:** Another theory put forward is 'Auto immune' theory. This happens when the immune system mistakenly seems to turn against the body. Normally in a healthy individual, antibodies are produced against the invading antigens, to protect the body. If the antibodies are directed against parts of the person's own body cells, they are called auto-antibodies and the disease is termed 'auto immune'. Thus the continued presence of many immune complexes initiates inflammation.

3. **Genetic Factor:** One can also inherit RA from his parents, grand parents. The hereditary traits produced by genes are called 'Genetic markers'.

Further Development of RA

In most cases, RA starts gradually spreading over several weeks with persistent pain and stiffness in one or more joints. Usually the hands and feet are first affected. This stiffness is worse on waking in the morning and wears off during the day. Later the arthritis may spread to other joints such as elbows, shoulders, hips, knees and ankles. Even the joints in the jaw and spine, especially the neck can be affected. Rarely a hoarse voice may indicate arthritis in the joints of larynx (voice box). At some stage the tendon sheaths frequently become inflammed which adds to the pain and swelling. Sometimes the fingers in hands and toes in the feet bend and deform in which case it becomes difficult to straighten that part.

RA is not only a disease of the joints. The whole body suffers. The person feels tired, weak, feverish. The muscles near the painful joint start getting smaller and this makes the weakness worse. Organs like lungs, heart, eyes and digestive system may also get involved in later stages.

Treatment of RA

Treatment consists of adequate rest, individually tailored exercise and physiotherapy, joint protection and suitable medication to control symptoms. Surgical procedures may be needed as an inevitable part of rehabilitation, to reduce the inflammatory symptoms and to promote routine activities, if so warranted by the situation.

Useful operations in rheumatoid arthritis are, median nerve decompression at the wrist, arthrodesis of wrist or ankles, synovectomy especially of the wrist and knee, repair of ruptured tendons, hip, knee and other joint replacement.

The objectives of drug therapy are to relieve pain, reduce inflammation, prevent deformities and to keep the joints functioning as effectively as possible.

Depending upon the intensity of the symptoms and signs, a qualified physician may administer the patient with Salicylates, NSAID (non-steroidal anti-inflammatory drugs), DMARDS (disease modifying anti-rheumatic drugs) such as gold salts, D-penicillamine, antimalarials and immunosupressive agents. Miscellaneous drugs such as tranquilizers, antidepressants, antibiotics, iron tablets, muscle relaxants are prescribed by physicians depending upon the symptoms.

Systemic corticosteroid therapy is usually given to in-patients who have not responded to other medications. An orthopaedic surgeon may decide to inject a steroid medicine to the affected joint with persistent inflammation, not responding to other medicines.

About one third of 'RA' patients have a mild illness with a high rate of spontaneous remission. Another third of the patients progress slowly with minor functional disability while the remaining have a significantly aggressive disease with only limited periods of partial or complete remission.

Except for infective arthritis, the disease seldom poses an emergency, therefore, surgical help for arthritis is considered the last resort. Severe arthritis which has caused extensive damage to the joints may call for surgery but otherwise drugs and rehabilitation can take care of the rest.

Osteoarthritis (OA)

It is the most common type of arthritis. It is a degenerative joint disease or wear and tear arthritis. It is the most common and oldest disease to affect humans. Most persons past the age of sixty have osteoarthritis to a lesser or higher degree.

Changes in the Joint in OA: In a healthy joint, the joint tissues (cartilages) are flexible and elastic, which help in smooth movement of joint. In OA, joint pathology is characterized by overgrowth of bone on one hand and loss of cartilage on the other. In OA, the cartilage gradually wears away leaving the ends of the bones unprotected. Without the proper gliding surface, the joint becomes painful to move.

The bone ends become thickened due to the formation of spurs of bone called 'osteophytes'. Bits of bone and cartilage may float loosely in the joint space and may contribute to pain which occurs with movement. At its worst, when the cartilage becomes completely worn out, the bone ends then grind painfully together when joint moves. The surounding tendons, ligaments and muscles are indirectly affected and become weaker.

Referred Pain in OA: Rarely the pain is felt far from the affected joint. This is known as 'referred pain' in Medical parlance. Some people with OA in their hips feel referred pain in their knees. OA of the spine can cause pressure on nerves that will cause pain in the arms or legs.

Joints Involved in OA: OA can occur in any joint. The weight bearing joints such as those of the hips, knees, feet and spine are the joints most often involved. The bones of the neck and the lower back are also commonly affected. Rarely affected joints are the wrists, elbows, ankles and finger joints which may get involved as a result of injuries or unusual stress.

Chondromalacia patella is a type of OA where there is a softening and loss of integrity of the knee cap or patella. People who have this problem may give a history of the knee cap slipping out of place. They may complain of pain in the knee joint which becomes worse after climbing stairs or after an unaccustomed physical activity.

Causes of OA: OA is divided into two broad categories:

1. **Primary OA:** In this type, degenerative changes occur in an otherwise normal joint. Primary OA is inherited also.

2. **Secondary OA:** In this type, the most common factor is thought to be faulty or excessive stress on joints. If a joint is deformed or dislocated, the perfect mating or matching of the cartilage surfaces is lost and OA develops. Similarly if a fracture is not properly set, the bones heal badly and the nearby joint is put to abnormal stress, which eventually produces OA.

Thus workers in certain occupations are more likely to develop degenerative changes in their joints because of unequal or excessive stressing of a joint e.g. the elbows in pneumatic drill workers, the knees in coal miners and the back of those lifting heavy weights. Even athletes and other players in certain sports appear to develop OA more commonly if they fail to let an injured joint heal properly before using it again. Obesity may also lead to secondary osteoarthritis in the weight bearing joints.

Investigations Required in Case of OA: Routine Blood tests, urine analysis, blood biochemistry and X-rays of the affected joint are usually advised.

X-rays findings of OA are narrowing of the joint space, presence of bone cysts surrounding the joint. CT scan and MRI may be required in patients in whom symptoms point to involvement of spine an narrowing of spinal column.

Symptoms of OA: The most common symptom is a nagging ache or painful feeling in the affected joints. They may be difficult to move and feel a little stiff. Usually these symptoms develop gradually over several months in middle aged or elderly people. A common complaint is that aching is worse during cold and damp weather. A common form of osteoarthritis, particularly in women involves the joints of the fingers, where knobbly lumps called "Heberden's nodes" appear at the side of the end joints and knuckles. Several fingers may become involved, causing pain and general discomfort. Also the pain increases after injury to the joint which may swell up with fluid. Overuse makes these symptoms worse. However, the pain and stiffness settle with rest and treatment.

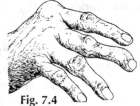

Fig. 7.4
Deformation of finger joints due to arthritis

In long standing cases, muscle wasting and joint deformity may also occur.

Difference between OA & RA

1. OA is essentially a condition of the joints and doesn't cause a general feeling of ill health, fever, poor appetite or weight loss. In this sense, therefore it is entirely different from RA in which the whole body suffers.

2. OA is more commonly associated with heavily stressed joints of lower limbs e.g. lower spine, hips, knees, ankles. But RA can occur anywhere in the body.

3. OA is age related and advances with ageing. RA is not age related. It can happen even to children.

4. In RA, normally symmetrical joints on both sides of the body are involved but in OA it is not necessary.

Treatment of OA: Please see the nature cure treatments given at the end of this chapter.

Ankylosing Spondylitis

It is a form of arthritis that essentially affects the spine and leads to stiffness of the back. 'Ankylosing' means stiff, 'spondyl' refers to spine; 'Itis' means inflammation. Hence this disease may be called inflammation and arthritis of the joints of the spinal bones (vertebrae) that tend to become stiff, rigid and fused together (ankylosis). It often occurs in young persons, and in extreme cases can result in a total stiffness of the spine as the bones fuse together, although the disease usually stops before this stage, leaving a stiff lower back and hips.

Cause: Research has shown that hereditary factors are very important. A gene type or genetic marker called HLA-B27 has been recently discovered in nearly 95% of the patients with ankylosing spondylitis. This means that someone with this B27 marker has a higher chance of developing this type of spondylitis.

Symptoms: The first symptom is pain and stiffness in lower back that is worse in the morning on waking up. The backache is due to imflammation of the sacroiliac joints (joints between the base of the spine (sacrum) and the hip bones). The inflammation gradually spreads up the spine (lumbar and dorsal) and even the neck may be stiff. If ignored and treatment is not done, the spine may begin to curve prominently. The affected joints tend to get fused and can eventually restrict a person's movements.

Diagnosis: The doctor is able to confirm the diagnosis by X-rays of the sacroiliac joints and spine, which will usually show the typical changes. He may also advise blood tests to look for the B27 marker.

Treatment: Exercise forms the mainstay of treatment. Rest appears to lead to increasing stiffness and fusion of joints.

Acute phase of the disease is controlled with non-steroidal anti-inflammatory drugs. Breathing exercises, spinal extension, flexion and rotation exercises are taught by a physiotherapist.

Genetic counselling may help to prevent the occurrence of the disease in future generations. In severally incapacitated patient, corrective surgery may be warranted.

Arthritis Associated with Rheumatic Fever

Rheumatic fever is an inflammatory syndrome which follows an inadequately treated or neglected infection of throat by a group of organisms called 'Beta haemolytic streptococci'.

Who is Susceptible to Rheumatic Fever?

Children aged 5 to 15 years and young adults are mostly affected by streptococcal sore throat and rheumatic fever.

Course of the Disease: Child comes first with a sore throat or cold, followed by an attack of tonsillitis or perhaps scarlet fever. While he is recovering from infection, one or two of his larger joints become red, swollen and tender to touch. There is also soreness in the muscles and tendons as well as lack of appetite and a feeling of weakness. Nose bleeding is common in rheumatic fever without any apparent outward cause.

Development of Arthritis in Rheumatic Fever: Normally larger joints are involved e.g. knee, ankles, elbows. Each joint is affected for a week or so but the process is migratory, shifting from one joint to another, with some overlap at times. Even as one joint improves, the next becomes inflammed. There is redness, swelling, local warmth in the affected joint and the patient is unable to move the joint. The arthritis of rheumatic fever heals very well if early action is taken by giving proper medications.

Effect on Heart: The real serious part of this disease is the damage it does to the valves of the heart. Certain streptococcus germs present in the throat are apparently responsible. The body becomes highly sensitized to their presence and it is this allergic response that harms. Although rheumatic fever affects the heart as a whole, the serious permanent damage occurs in the valves, most frequently the mitral and aortic valves. ECG and X-ray of the heart can indicate the damage to heart done uptil now.

Treatment: Rheumatic fever can usually be prevented by treating sore throats or other streptococcal infections properly. Penicillin is still the best medicine for severe sore throats. It helps to clear out the haemolytic streptococcus germs from the throat. If patient is sensitive to penicillin, tetracycline or other medication prescribed by physician can be given. Patients who have had rheumatic fever may have to take these medication for a long time.

Juvenile Chronic Arthritis (JCA)

This mostly occurs in children of less than 16 years and tends to last for a long time.

Diagnostic Criteria for JCA

1. Age of onset less than 16 years
2. Arthritis in one or more joints with limitation of range of motion, pain on moving the joint and increased temperature over the affected joint.
3. Duration of disease—6 weeks to 3 months
4. Disease may be polyarthritis (involving 5 joints or more), oligo arthritis (involving 4 joints or more) or in the form of a systemic disease (arthritis, intermittent fever, rheumatoid rash, enlarged liver, spleen and lymph nodes).
5. Other types of arthritis have to be excluded.

Tests for Diagnosis: ESR, RF-test, ANF, synovial fluid aspirations and examinations are a few tests routinely carried out to confirm the diagnosis.

Treatment: Aspirin is the drug of choice which is well tolerated in children with JCA, NSAID and immunomodulators are also prescribed at the discretion of physician. Doctors usually avoid administering corticosteroid drugs in treating JCA because of the side effects such as growth retardation, softening of bones, reduced resistance to infection, High B.P. Once the inflammation is controlled, active physiotherapy must be started. Irreversibly damaged joints may have to be treated by surgery, once the child reaches an appropriate age.

Infective Arthritis

Joint infections can occur due to infectious organisms such as bacteria (staphylococcus), viruses, mycobacteria (as in tuberculosis), spirochaets (as in syphilis). Joint infection can also occur indirectly as a result of infection elsewhere in the body by **steptococci (as in rheumatic fever) or due to sexually transmitted diseases such as gonorrhea or AIDS.** HIV (human immuno deficiency virus), responsible for causing AIDS has also been recovered in synovial fluid with acute arthritis. HIV-related infective arthritis may be present along with a co-infection, such as Reiter's Syndrome and Psoriatic arthritis.

Symptoms are a single hot joint, pain and inflammation are present in the joint and the skin surrounding it is warm and red. Patient may be suffering from fever, chills and weakness. The joint which is affected is often a knee, shoulder, hip, ankle or wrist. In some cases, more than one joint may get infected.

Alcoholics, drug abusers, persons who have diabetes, kidney disease, some forms of cancer are more likely candidates than the average person, for infective arthritis.

Antibiotics are the usual treatment for joint infections caused by bacteria.

Aspiration and examination of the synovial fluid of the infected joint will help the doctor to diagnose the organisms causing infection. If an untreated 'staphylococcus' infection is present, an orthopaedic surgeon may open and drain the joint surgically, remove damaged tissue, and irrigate the area thoroughly, remove damaged tissue, and irrigate the area thoroughly. The infection is then treated **by delivering the antibiotics directly to the joint via fine catheters** (tubes).

Arthritis may also be a consequence of mumps, German measles, hepatitis-B virus infection (jaundice). All these are self limiting and arthritis disappears when the infection gets dissolved completely.

Gout

This is a type of arthritis that has been known since the time of the Greeks and Romans. It mainly affects the men after the age of 40 and is unusual in women, except those past the menopause.

Cause: Gout is caused by crystals of uric acid forming particularly in the joints, kidneys and as stones in the urinary tract. Uric acid is one of the end products of the body's chemical processes. Victims of gout have a higher level of uric acid in the blood than normal either due to increased amount being formed or reduced amount of acid being passed out by the kidneys into the urine. In human beings, more than 70% of uric acid is excreted through the urine and rest through the digestive system. The uric acid normally remains dissolved in the blood but when there is an excess of uric acid in the blood, the uric acid forms needle shaped crystals in the joints which bring about an attack of gout. Uric acid crystals may also get deposited in kidney and as stones in urinary tract.

An acute attack of gouty arthritis can be triggered by crash diets, injury to a joint, excessive intake of alcohol, eating too much meats, sweet breads, mushrooms, cauliflower and peas. *In fact foods rich in 'purines' which the body converts into uric acid (such as liver, kidney, meat extracts, sardines and fish roe (including caviar) and certain drinks such as port, burgundy* and other red wines may contribute to a person developing gout

Symptoms: The big toe is usually the first to get affected by the disease. The toe may become acutely painful, tender, hot and swollen in a sudden attack and the sufferer may be awakened in the middle of night, having gone to bed happily the night before. Without treatment, the acute attack subsides over one or two weeks. Between the attacks, the person usually feels no symptoms. Repeated attacks can damage the involved joints.

When gout has been present for a long time, urate crystals get deposited under the skin (over the elbow, on the outer edge of the ear) or near affected joints. If gout is not treated, these deposits or Tophi may break through the skin and become infected. Heel, ankle, other joints of the feet, knee, wrist, fingers and elbow may also get infected. If the disease progresses, deformities can occur from inflammatory destruction of the joint structure. It is also to be noted that probability of gout patients developing uric acid stones is far greater than persons without gout.

Tests required to be done: Before starting treatment, the doctor may desire the following tests to be done:

1. Blood test to measure the uric acid
2. X-ray
3. Fluid from the affected joint is aspirated and examined under a microscope in order to establish the presence of urate crystals.

Treatment: Medication for gout consists of three types of drugs.

i. **Colchicine and certain NSAID's** control the inflammation of a gouty attack.

ii. A second category is called **uricosuric agents** which increase the body's ability to eliminate uric acid in urine, thus lowering the amount of uric acid in the blood. 'Probenecid' and 'Sulfinpyrazone' are the two commonly used uricosuric drugs.

iii. The third category of antigout drug i.e. **'Allopurinol'** decreases uric acid levels in the blood by reducing the rate at which the body produces uric acid.

A person having gout is also required to avoid or restrict eating certain foods such as meat, fish, sardines, sweet breads, yeast, cauliflower, mushrooms, spinach, peas which contain moderate or high purine content.

Pseudogout

It is also known as CPPD disease (Calcium Pyro Phosphate Dihydrate Crystal deposition disease). This disease affects elderly people above the age of 60, both men and women and occurs due to deposition of calcium crystals in the joints. Pain and swellings may be prominent in wrists and fingers as well as the knee.

Many causes have been attributed to pseudogout. Over activity of parathyroid glands cause too much calcium to build up in the body, which may get deposited as crystals in the joints. Decreased thyroid glands activity can also lead to CPPD disease.

For diagnosis of the disease, Doctor will advise blood tests for thyroid and parathyroid functions along with X-ray and assess blood calcium and phosphorus level.

Joint aspiration, medication, rest, special exercise and protection of the joints are advised to control the symptoms and retain good function of the affected joints.

Some Nature Cure Remedies for Treatment of Arthritis

1. **Contrast Hydrotherapy:** It has an exhilarating benefit upon the sluggish metabolic and circulatory system. Apply first hot pack at the joint for a few minutes. Now apply cold pack on the joint. Duration of hot pack should be more than cold pack. It increases the blood circulation through the joint tremendously.

2. **Body Brushing:** Bath brush with stiff bristles are available in the market. Rub yourself with this brush all over with special attention on the affected joint. This invigorates the whole circulatory system of the body and the toxins are flushed away from the joint reducing the pain in the joint. If brush is not available, you can also do the rubbing with your dry towel.

3. **Massage:** Massage around the affected joint is very useful to reduce pain in the aching joint. It speeds up the blood circulation and relaxes tight muscles around the joint. Just rub or stroke gently around the joint and press around the

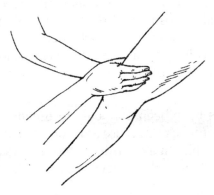

Fig. 7.5 Massage around knee joint

128

joint using fingers and thumb. It is important not to hack or pound or use forceful movements over arthritic joint. Massage can be done preferably after applying some pain removing (Analgesic) oil or cream (e.g. Rheumatil Oil or Gel of M/s. Dabur).

4. **Heat Treatment:** The best way to give heat is dipping the affected joint in hot water contained in a vessel or bucket. Salt can also be mixed in it. You can also subject the affected joint to hot bath and hot shower while bathing. Heat improves the circulation around the joint and relaxes the surrounding muscles. Heat can also be applied by hot water bottle or an electrical heating pad or infrared lamp.

5. **Exercises:** The most important treatment for controlling arthritis is exercise. Exercises for arthritics must cover all the following three types:

   i. **Endurance exercises** e.g. aerobics like, walking, jogging, running, swimming etc. However those types of aerobic exercises should be chosen which don't provide direct impact or stress to the affected joint otherwise a weak joint can get further damaged.

   ii. **Stretching exercises** which move the joint as far as it will comfortably go in all possible directions and then coaxing it to go a little further in every subsequent attempts just beyond the point where pain begins. Some of the joint movement exercises are shown below:

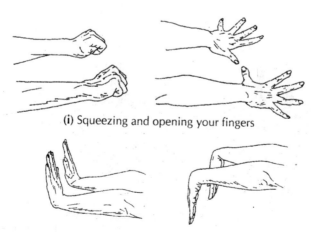

(i) Squeezing and opening your fingers

(ii) Wrist bending

Fig. 7.6 (Contd...)

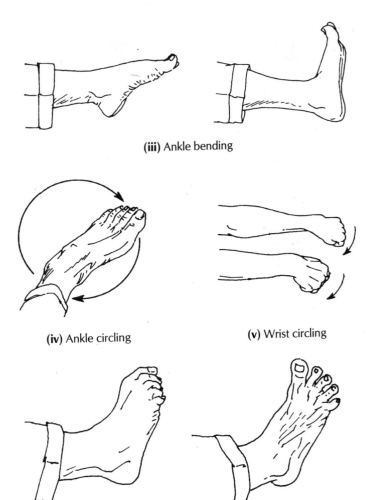

(iii) Ankle bending

(iv) Ankle circling   **(v)** Wrist circling

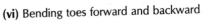

(vi) Bending toes forward and backward

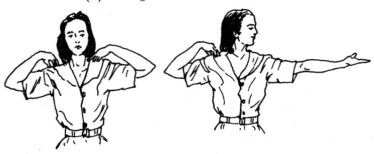

(vii) Elbow bending: arms at the sides

Fig. 7.6 (Contd...)

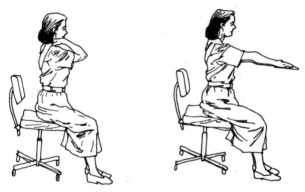

(viii) Elbow bending: arms forward

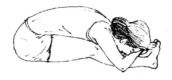

(ix) Stretching exercise to increase blood circulation in entire
leg so as to reduce arthritis in hips, knee and ankles

Fig. 7.6

iii. **Muscle strengthening exercises:** By increasing muscle
strength, stability is imparted to the vulnerable joint and
more load can be shared by the muscle even if the joint
has degenerated.

Exercise nourishes cartilages and builds strong tissues.
Cartilages in a joint have only one source of nourishment
i.e. from synovial fluid. This fluid can enter the joint only
through exercise. Without movement the synovial
membrane gradually adheres to the joint cartilage like
scotch tape. Eventually it obscures the joint so that the
cartilage can't get nutrition and quietly begins to
degenerate.

Joints must be used otherwise they will get frozen and
become immobile and muscles and tendons associated
with them will get weak and bones softer. The saying **'Use
it or lose it'** is very true.

However it is advisable to keep the following things in
mind before exercising:

a. Don't exercise a joint when it is inflammed and painful. Allow it to rest and apply hot and cold fomentation to it.

b. You should start with slow and gentle movements and little warm up. It may be advisable to have a massage before exercise or having a hot shower or bath before exercise. Then have a slow stretch and movement to begin with and gradually increase the limit of stretching.

c. Every time you should go slightly beyond the point when it starts to pain but only slightly because if you try to force too much, you may tear your tendons and muscles.

a. Muscle strengthening exercises are as important as joint movement and flexibility exercises. Below is shown one such exercise to strengthen the muscles around knee joint (quadriceps muscle). This is very helpful to tackle the arthritis of knee joint. Here you sit on a table. Keep a load (preferably a bag full of sand) on the upper side of your foot. Now straighten your knee with this load and then bring back your leg to normal bent position. Do it several times. (see fig. 7.7).

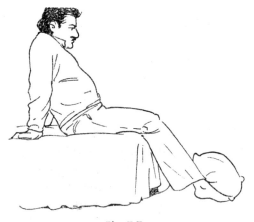

Fig. 7.7

The key point in strengthening the muscles associated with a joint is that you open or move a joint against a resisting force by using your muscles without any direct pressure on the joint. You can also strengthen your quadriceps by tightening and releasing your quadriceps off and on without any load on the foot with straight leg position while sitting, lying or standing position as shown in the following figure.

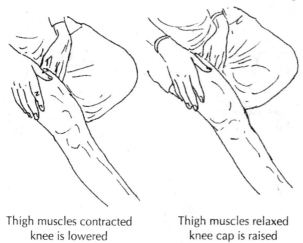

Thigh muscles contracted
knee is lowered

Thigh muscles relaxed
knee cap is raised

Fig. 7.7A

Keeping these principles in mind, one can strengthen muscles across any joint.

6. **Passive Stretching:** Passive stretching of joint by someone else is also helpful for unlocking the joint and increasing the blood circulation. There should be only slight jerk to be given for stretching the joint and sudden uncontrolled jerks with too much force should be avoided. Below is shown the passive movement and stretching of hip joint. Keeping the leg straight, slowly raise it as far as it will comfortably go and then stretch.

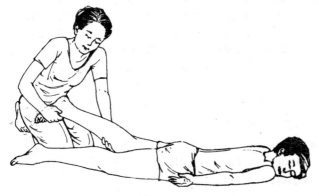

Fig. 7.8

133

Similarly, so many other passive movements can be given to the joints of an arthritic person. Some of them are shown below:

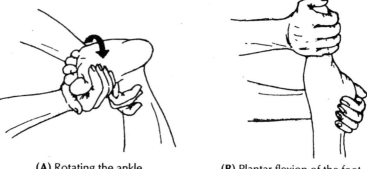

(A) Rotating the ankle   (B) Plantar flexion of the foot

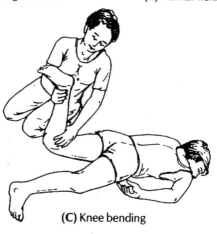

(C) Knee bending

Fig. 7.9

7. **Sunbathing:** Controlled sunbathing is most soothing to the arthritics. The sunshine activates small glands beneath the surface of the skin to manufacture vitamin D, which is used by the metabolism to help strengthen weak or porous bones and build resistance to arthritis. Sunshine also facilitates better calcium absorption.

   Hence, try to have one hour of sunshine everyday outdoor during a good sunshine weather.

8. **Garlic:** Garlic and Fenugreek ('Methi') are said to have anti-arthritic property. Hence, try to include these in your dietary habits. Garlic tablets are also available in the market.

9. **Reduction in Body Weight:** Obesity is closely associated with osteoarthritis because more weight implies more stress on the joints especially of lower limbs (hips, knees, ankle). Hence, all steps should be taken to reduce the weight of the body if a person is overweight.

10. **Vayu Mudra:** There is one mudra called 'Vayu Mudra' which is helpful in diseases relating to Arthritis. In this mudra, index finger is placed at the base of thumb and pressed lightly with the thumb. It can be done many times whenever you feel convenient.

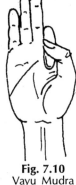
Fig. 7.10
Vayu Mudra

11. **Ice Treatment:** Applying ice on the swollen and painful joints of arthritis also gives relief. But, ice should not be applied directly. It should be applied after keeping it in some plastic bag.

12. **Acupressure:** For arthritis in hip joints, knee joints, ankle joints, giving acupressure at the following places is found quite useful.

   i. **Around Ankles:** Give pressure around all the four ankle bones in both the legs. Pressing the back of heel and achilli tendons as shown in Fig. 7.12 is quite helpful for reducing knee joint pain.

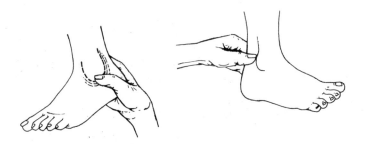

Figs. 7.11   **Figs. 7.12**

   ii. Give pressure on the back of legs at the following points as shown in the figure.

   a. In the middle of knee

   b. Outside of hips

   c. At the bottom of hips in the middle

135

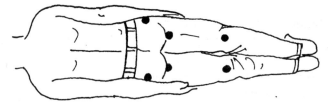

Fig. 7.13

You can also do deep pressure massage on the whole back of leg right from ankle to hips. It will automatically press these acupressure points.

iii. Give pressure on the palms and soles at the points shown in the figure either in the form of massage or separate pointed pressure. These points are specially useful for reducing knee pain.

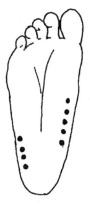

Fig. 7.14

iv. Give pressure on a point located at the junction of knee and inner side of leg as shown in the figure. This is also useful in reducing knee pain.

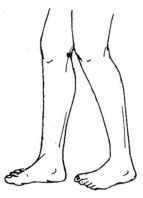

For exact location of these acupressure points, feeling of sensitivity/ tenderness/pain is the guide by which you can exactly identify them.

Fig. 7.15

Diet for Arthritic Patient

An arthritic should observe following dietary regulations:

a. Increase water consumption to 8 or more glasses a day.

b. All foods as much as possible should be eaten fresh, raw and natural. Fruits and vegetables should be consumed in plenty.

c. Eliminate tobacco, alcohol, refined carbohydrates, saturated fats, fried foods, parantha, meat, tea, coffee, cold items, icecream, rice, sugar, sweetmeats, processed and canned foods.

d. Take vitamins, minerals, enzymes in enough quantity. Vitamin C, D, E, B-complex and in minerals calcium, iodine and copper are particularly good for arthritics.

e. Avoid those eatables which increase **'vayu'** or **'vata'** dosha in the body e.g. cauliflower, ladyfinger (Bhindi), colocesia (Arbi), Red pumpkin gourd (Kashifal), Brinjal (Bangan), Urad dal, Rajma, potato, rice and its products, sour food (e.g. curd, curry, raita etc.).

Some Useful Practical Suggestions

i. Don't wear shoes with high heels. These cause poor posture, shorten the calf muscles and hamstrings. High heeled shoes put excessive weight on the forward part of the foot. Similarly a shoe with narrow toes makes the foot muscles rigid and tense. This upsets circulation and precipitates arthritic distress.

ii. Wear comfortable socks. If they are too tight they interfere with the relaxation of your toes and feet and cause congestion leading to arthritic pain.

iii. Your collars should always be comfortably loose. A collar that is too tight or too high can cause a stiff neck, a form of arthritis in this area.

iv. You should sleep on a firm mattress which doesn't sag.

v. Many people develop arthritic pains because of faulty reading positions. When you read in an awkward position, you cause neck and back sprain by forcing your muscles in an unnatural position. This congestion interferes with free circulation and may result in neck and shoulder arthritis. One shouldn't hunch or slump also while reading.

vi.   Prolonged driving can cause congestion of the musculoskeletal system and impede a free circulation. One shouldn't drive more than one or two hours at a stretch. Stop as often as you can. Get out walk around, shake your hands. Shake your legs. Shrug your shoulders. This way you will protect yourself against arthritis flare up.

Further while driving, sit close to your steering wheel so your knees are comfortably bent. Don't slump forward.

vii.   Many persons find it difficult to get up after sitting in one position for an hour or more. This indicates a sluggish circulation with arthritic-like painful symptoms. If you know you have to sit for a certain period of time, schedule regular walking breaks. As often as possible, get up, move around, limber up your muscles. Shrug your shoulders. You know which parts of your body are tense, so shake them and loosen up the muscles of your neck and back. Wobble your head from side to side.

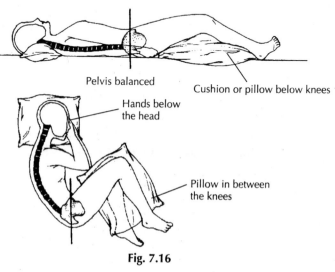

Pelvis balanced

Cushion or pillow below knees

Hands below the head

Pillow in between the knees

Fig. 7.16

138

viii. Don't sleep over the stomach as it increases the hollow in your lower back and creates strain in your musculoskeletal system. Sleep on your back. Keep knees propped up over a cushion. Or else sleep on your side with knees comfortably bent and drawn up. This keeps your pelvis and spine in a balanced and comfortable position as shown in the figure and doesn't cause any stress on these joints.

ix. Reduce emotional stress as it is an important precipitating factor in arthritis. Emotional stress exerts a control on the glands of internal secretion, particularly the thyroid, adrenal and pituitary and these glands play an important role in the bone and joint metabolism.

x. Gradually decrease all drugs to the minimum by following nature cure treatments. Reduce and slowly eliminate all corticosteroid medications.

xi. Arthritics should take sufficient rest and a rushing life style should be totally avoided.

xii. Don't allow the joints to remain still for long periods. Occasionally get up to stretch the joints to prevent stiffness.

xiii. Do occasional balancing exercises on both sides of the body which will help the joints to come into good relationship with each other and improve the posture. Two such exercises are shown below:

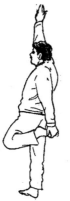 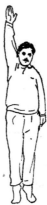

Fig. 7.17 Do with both legs alternately   **Fig. 7.18** Stretching each hand up and down alternately, standing on your toes

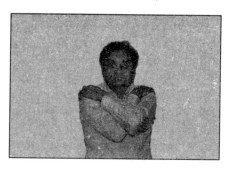

Fig. 7.19 Place hands on the opposite shoulders

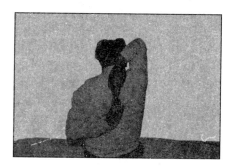

Fig. 7.20 Reach around and behind back with left hand. Bring right hand from above the shoulder and try to touch fingers of both the hands. Then reverse the position of hands and do the same on other shoulder.

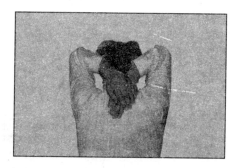

Fig. 7.21 Put one hand over the other over the middle of upper back (back of Thymus). Keep yor head straight and look in front. This is important for proper posture.

8. Peptic Ulcer

What is Peptic Ulcer

Peptic ulcer is the term designated for localized destruction of the inner wall or mucosa of the stomach (called gastric ulcer) or the upper part of the small intestine (called duodenal ulcer). In other words, it is a wound inside the stomach or duodenum. The term 'Peptic ulcer' can be used to describe both a stomach/gastric ulcer or a duodenal ulcer. Peptic ulcer is usually associated with hyperacidity.

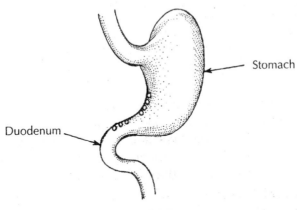

Fig. 8.1

Duodenal ulcer is the commonest and seems to occur especially in men; and gastric or stomach ulcer, tends to attack both men and women. According to latest survey about one in ten people will have an ulcer at some time in an average span of life.

What Causes Peptic Ulcer

We all know that when food comes into stomach for digestion, stomach produces various gastric juices of which the most important is hydrochloric acid. In the process of ulceration, this acid starts eating the lining of stomach/duodenum. Ulcers of all kinds result from an imbalance between the power of the stomach's acid secretions to attack and the ability of the stomach/duodenal lining to resist the attack.

This is the reason that some people who have more acid secretion don't suffer from ulceration, while others who have low acidity may have peptic ulcer. Hence we can say that susceptibility to peptic ulcer depends on two factors:

1. Factors which increase acid secretion in stomach e.g. hot and spicy food, fatty foods, excessive smoking, excessive use of alcohol, tea, coffee and certain drugs like corticosteroids, caffeine, reserpine etc.
2. Weakness of lining or mucosa of stomach/duodenum to resist the attack of acid.

   Hence obviously to deal with ulcer, it is usually necessary to either increase the resistance of the mucosa or decrease the production of acid.

Symptoms of Peptic Ulcer

An ulcer is associated with a sharp, penetrating and burning type of pain in the upper part of the abdomen. Since symptoms of gastric ulcer and duodenal ulcer differ, let us describe them separately:

i. **Gastric Ulcer:** Gastric ulcer pain is usually localized to the epigastrium, a central point about half way between the chin and the umbilicus and eating usually makes it worse. Unlike duodenal ulcer pain, gastric ulcer pain doesn't usually go away once it has started.

ii. **Duodenal Ulcer:** The pain in duodenal ulcer is also localized in the epigastrium and unlike gastric ulcers, eating usually helps relieve the pain. Another point of difference is that while in gastric ulcers, the pain is increased immediately after the meal, in duodenal ulcers it may take 2 to 3 hours time. Another characteristic factor of duodenal ulcer is that it tends to disappear for weeks or even months at a time for no apparent reason.

One may ask as to why there is pain following meals. This is due to the stimulation of acid secretion which flows over the ulcer stimulating the pain receptor. In duodenal ulcer, it takes about 2 to 3 hours time for the acid to reach the site of ulcer which explains the reason for delay in occurrence of pain in these patients.

Diagnosis of Ulcer

Diagnosis consists of X-ray after a barium meal. Actual examination of the stomach and its contents can also be done by a process known as **'Endoscopy'**. Biopsy can also be done in the process to ascertain the actual condition.

Stress and Ulcer

Stress is one of the important factors to cause ulcer in your stomach. Stress increases the flow of acid in your stomach. This extra acid that flows into your stomach is designed to turn any food there into digestible form as soon as possible. But with no food to work on, this acid erodes the lining of the stomach and produces an ulcer.

Treatment of Peptic Ulcer

The treatment of peptic ulcer consists of general measures which include control of diet and other lifestyle changes and use of specific drugs. If complications like bleeding or perforation at the site of ulcer occur, surgical intervention may become necessary. In an acute peptic ulcer, the treatment mainly consists of milk given at 15 minutes to 2 hours interval, depending on the severity of illness, for a week, along with drugs. *Milk not only counteracts acidity but also delays the emptying time of the stomach to allow the drugs to act for a longer period. An ulcer generally heals in 4 to 6 weeks of treatment.*

General Nature Cure Treatment

Most important factor in nature cure treatment is control of diet and develop good eating habits. Persons having ulcer had better avoid or reduce the foods given in the list below:

1. All fried foods
2. Strong tea or coffee

3. Fizzy drinks

4. Alcohol

5. Tobacco/smoking (Tobacco irritates the lining of the stomach and makes it more vulnerable to attack by acid)

6. Fatty foods

7. Spicy foods

8. Pickles, curry, peppers, mustard

9. Unripe fruit

10. Broad beans, brussels sprouts, radishes and cucumber

11. Very hot or very cold foods

12. Coarse bread, biscuits or cereals

13. Nuts or dried fruits

14. Any tough food (e.g. meat) that can't be chewed easily.

It is not necessary to avoid all these foods completely. You can find out which foods upset you more and you can avoid them.

Further you should develop good eating habits e.g.

1. Eat slowly, don't make hurry in eating

2. Don't eat while reading or watching T.V. Concentrate on eating

3. Don't put huge amount of food into your mouth at one time. Put small amount of food at one time and chew it properly before swallowing

4. Taste and relish each mouthful of food. This will increase the digestibility of food

5. Eat only when hungry

6. Try to have regular meals so that acid secretion is regularized

7. Don't do heavy physical work after eating.

Other important factor in nature cure is reduction of mental stress and anxiety and learning to lead a relaxed life. Since stress management is itself a vast topic in itself, reader may study separate books on this subject.

Drugs in Peptic Ulcer

In the acute stage of disease, use of drugs is a necessity and one can't solely rely on diet control but after reaching to a stable condition, one should gradually reduce the use of drugs and rely more and more on nature cure treatments as drugs can't cure the root cause of the problem and create many side effects. The drugs used in the treatment of peptic ulcer are mainly of the following kinds. These are prescribed by the doctor after carefully assessing the condition of the patient.

1. Drugs which counteract the acid secreted in the stomach e. g. Antacids
2. Drugs which inhibit acid secretion e.g. Ranitidine, Cimetidine, Famotidine, Rexatidine etc.
3. Drugs which delay food emptying from the stomach e.g. Anticholinergic drugs
4. Drugs which promote ulcer healing e.g. Omeprazole
5. Drugs providing protection to Mucosa e.g. Sucralfate, Misoprostol, Carbenoxalone etc.
6. Drugs which reduce anxiety and stress e.g. tranquilizers like diazepam (calmpose). These drugs are required to be given when patient shows high level of anxiety and stress. But they should be used for a short period because they lead to habituation and addiction.

A Few Words about Antacids

Since antacids are very frequently used in problems of acidity, it will be worthwhile to give more details about this for a layman.

Antacids counteract the effect of acid in the stomach mainly to provide symptomatic relief and to a lesser extent to promote healing of ulcer. It must be emphasized that the stomach keeps on emptying itself and the action of antacid lasts only for a shortwhile, irrespective of the dose taken. It is therefore important to take an antacid at frequent intervals or to adopt measures which delay the emptying of the stomach. Increasing the dose doesn't prolong the antacid action appreciably. Food delays emptying, prolonging the duration of action of antacids.

Same is true for anticholinergic drugs and for this reason these are given with antacids. Antacids can be divided into two major groups, those absorbable from the intestines and those non-absorbable. Since absorbable antacids produce actions all over the body (systemic effect), non absorbable antacids are preferred.

Antacids are available as liquids, powders and tablets. Liquids and powders usually work better than tablets (which need to be chewed or sucked very slowly). But for carrying purpose tablets are more convenient. There is no need to seek medical advice before using antacids to obtain temporary relief.

Antacids like other medicines have side effects. The two commonest side effects are diarrhoea and constipation. Antacids with magnesium salts usually cause diarrhoea and Antacids with aluminium salts tend to cause constipation. To overcome these problems many manufacturers sell mixtures of both aluminium and magnesium salt. But antacids shouldn't be used persistently.

9. Constipation

Constipation is irregular or difficult bowel movements and delayed emptying of bowels. Before discussing constipation and its treatment it will be worthwhile to review our digestive system briefly so as to have better appreciation of this disease.

Digestive System of Body

The digestive process begins as soon as food enters the mouth. It is chewed and mixed with saliva and then it passes down the oesophagus. Saliva is secreted by Salivary Glands. The flow of saliva is regulated by nervous stimuli, which may result from the sight or smell of appetizing food. Normally a person secretes between one and one-and-a-half litres of saliva daily.

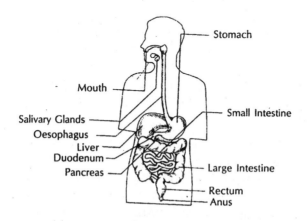

Fig. 9.1

147

From the oesophagus food goes to stomach. Stomach produces gastric juice which besides aiding in digestion, destroys most germs that might otherwise enter the intestine. The inner surface of the stomach is covered with mucous. A churning movement mixes food with gastric juice and reduces the food to a semi-liquid mass called **'Chyme'**. From the stomach, **'chyme'** enters duodenum where bile is added to it by liver and pancreatic juice is added to it by pancreas. Bile and pancreatic juices emulsify the fats and starches and convert them into assimilable form called **'Chyle'**.

Chyle is gradually carried along by waves of contraction until it reaches the small intestine. Here the food mixes with various enzymes and digestive fluids by a series of contractions of the intestinal wall. The contractions move the semi-liquid food back and forth in wave motions called *peristalsis.* All digestible food material is dissolved and absorbed here through tiny tubes called **Villi**, and digestion is complete.

Non-digestible portion of food goes to large intestine. When it reaches here, a great deal of the water is absorbed and ultimately the semisolid faeces are expelled from the body.

Large Intestine—the Site of Constipation

It is the large intestine or colon which is our major focus as far as the constipation is concerned. So let us elaborate its anatomy further.

After valuable portions of the food mass have been absorbed in small intestine, the balance—the waste or refuse passes through a small opening known as *Ileo-Caecal valve* into the colon. This little valve allows the waste to pass freely into the colon but prevents any of it from returning to small intestine.

The Caecum is a large blind end of the Colon, just beyond, the point where the waste enters it from the small intestine. It is a rounded cavity. The 'Appendix' attached to the Caecum is the little worm like appendage which when inflammed gives rise to the trouble known as 'Appendicitis'. It is from one to five inches in length and its function is still not very clear.

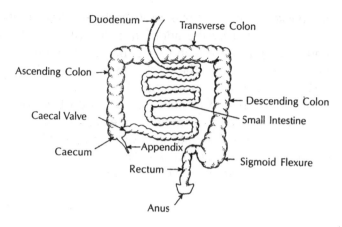

Fig. 9.2

Colon or large intestine is about 5 feet in length consisting mainly of the following parts:

1. Ascending Colon on right side of abdomen.
2. Transverse Colon over the small intestine.
3. Descending Colon on left side of abdomen.
4. Sigmoid flexure—A knotty shape twist or curve on lower left hand side of abdomen.
5. Rectum—Smaller tube below Sigmoid Flexure.
6. Anus—End part of Rectum. It is the outer rear opening through which the refuse passes from the body.

Mechanism of Constipation

So we have seen that the colon is the great sewer of body through which the waste matter (also known as the 'faeces') is carried away towards the anus. When this great sewer is allowed to become clogged, the condition called 'constipation' ensues accompanied by other evils associated with it.

The walls of the colon contain tiny absorbent channels which tend to reabsorb into the system the foul putrefying poisonous excrement which accumulates and chokes up the colon. It is like the action of a sewer which backs up into your house drain pipes when it becomes clogged.

Even if a person discharges everyday, still he may be constipated and may have a loaded colon. If from one end of this packed colon, a small quantity is discharged daily, the colon still remains full by the addition at the other end and thus constipation is present and continues even though there may be a daily discharge. The discharge is from the lower end of colon only. So daily movements of bowels are no sign that the colon is not loaded or constipated. Colon has got amazing capacity for holding excrement by extending and swelling of its walls. Investigation into the faecal matters of the colon of some badly constipated patients has sometimes revealed such a dry and hardened excrement so as to resist the knife. The mass may be so enormous as to press upon any organ located in the abdomen, interfering with its functions. It may also press liver arresting the flow of bile or urinary organs crippling their functions. The hardened faecal matter can eat into the sensitive mucous membrane, causing serious inflammation of the colon.

The most common part of the colon to become enlarged is the Sigmoid Flexure and the Caecum. Accumulations can occur in any part of the colon. The ascending colon is much

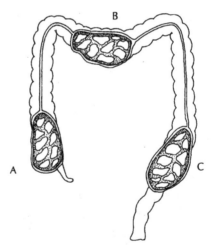

Fig. 9.3

Condition of a loaded colon in chronic constipation: Lumps of hard faeces accumulate either at A (caecum), B (middle of transverse colon) or C (sigmoid flexure). The colon enlarges at these parts and it becomes very difficult for the lumps to push their way on to be expelled. In trying to pass, they scratch the delicate membrane and produce the most excruciating pain of 'Colic'. If the accumulation is at 'B', the part of the colon sags producing good deal of discomfort and, at times, pain in the pit of stomach.

nore often filled than normally thought. Infact chronic accumulations are often to be found in the ascending colon than in the descending colon. When the accumulations are large, the increased weight of the colon tends to displace it and the transverse colon may descend even into the pelvis.

Causes of Constipation

The colon among the majority of animals and persons living a natural life is free from obstructions and is evacuated by frequent natural passages. However with the modern sedentary life style and unnatural habits, normal evacuations from the colon are disturbed.

The most important causes of constipation are a disregard of the call to pass motion and an improper diet. When the rectum is full it sends signals to the intestines through the Central Nervous System for their movement and if this is repeatedly ignored, it gradually leads to failure of the rectum to signal the urge.

In modern conditions, the rush to work place or school or to catch morning train may interfere with the habit of regular defecation. The sensation of the "call of nature" once voluntarily suppressed may not easily return again throughout the day. Moreover, many schools and offices are inadequately provided with necessary conveniences, and once the habit of regular defecation is broken, the person becomes constipated.

A diet with no roughage and fibres predisposes one to constipation. The diet should contain a reasonable amount of non-absorbable material or fibres to form a bulk which acts as a stimulus for the intestinal movements.

Highly spicy foodstuffs such as chaat, pickles and hot curries containing chillies and condiments may stimulate the bowel to cause a complete evacuation but this is followed by inactivity of the intestines and constipation. Alcohol, tea, coffee also act in just the same way. Similarly purgatives also stimulate the intestines to cause their evacuation and this is also followed by constipation. Foods which have little residue, such as meat, fish, eggs and cheese and especially a diet which is composed almost exclusively of milk, are often productive of troublesome constipation by failing to provide sufficient stimulus to the normal movement of intestines.

Other causes of constipation are mental stress, lack of exercise, lack of adequate water intake, abnormality of gastrointestinal tract, adverse effects of drugs, drying of stool (faecal impaction), obstruction of the intestines and severe illness in which food intake is too small.

Effect of Mental State on Bowel Movement

The influence of mind in causing constipation is quite common enough. Some persons cannot move their bowels when anxious or worried or in unusual surroundings. Failure to move bowels on the first day of a vacation or on visit to a new place, is usually due to the unfamiliar lavatory, and perhaps to the unusual hour of getting up; such small changes being sufficient to upset the nervous control of defecation. Workers on alternate day and night shifts are likewise at a disadvantage and may become very worried about failure of a previous regular habit.

The movements of colon may be more consistently impaired by the loss of muscle tone which is apt to occur with sedentary habits, and in old age too. Malnutrition, dropsy or melancholia and depression are also associated with inactivity of the colon.

Physical Symptoms of Constipation

Absorption of foul matter from the colon due to constipation leads to many outward physical symptoms which gives the clue about a person being constipated.

1. Yellow complexion
2. Dry and muddy skin
3. Furred tongue
4. Foul and fetid breath
5. Colour of faeces—A black or very dark green colour almost always indicates that the faeces are old. Prompt discharge of refuse is indicated by more or less yellow colour
6. Yellow eye balls
7. Strong sweaty exhalations

8. Indigestion, heart burn, Dyspepsia

9. Vertigo, Headache

Constipated patients invariably suffer from anaemia (bloodlessness).

Results of Chronic Constipation

The worst feature of an impacted or loaded colon is that it becomes the breeding place for innumerable germs of disease which are absorbed in the circulation and which are thus carried to all parts of the body poisoning and infecting the various organs.

When the Colon is clogged, it prevents the ordinary passage of the food through stomach and intestines. The food being retained in the stomach and small intestines far beyond its natural time, is apt to ferment and throw off acid substances which aid in poisoning the system generating gas and causing heart burn, sour stomach etc. The liver, kidneys and lungs can become infected and their action impaired.

Nature uses the kidneys and skin to eliminate as much of the impurity as possible but sooner or later the kidneys become overworked and broken down. The skin becomes muddy, foul and filled with eruptions.

In short a loaded colon brings about a condition of poisoned blood which actually creates crisis in the whole body .

Chronic constipation may eventually lead to the following dreaded diseases:

1. **Piles:** There are various veins in the rectum and around the anus. Piles are swollen veins around the anus. Constipation and straining is the main cause of the presence of piles. Piles occur both inside and outside the anus and can be painful and even bleed with excessive straining due to pressure on veins.

2. **Colitis:** Chronic ulcerative colitis is a severe prolonged inflammation of the colon or large bowel in which ulcers form in the wall of the colon, resulting in the passage of bloody stools mixed with pus and mucus. Chronic

ulcerative colitis usually begins in the lower part of the bowel and spreads upward.

3. Prolapse of rectum or hernia and anal fissure/fistula may also result due to straining during evacuation.

Treatment of Constipation

1. Never disregard the call for motion and don't wait unnecessarily. Rush to the toilet wherever you are.

2. Try to have a bowel movement at the same time each day devoting ten to fifteen minutes. However it is important to avoid straining.

3. One should drink from six to eight glasses of water each day. Drinking two glasses of water (preferably by mixing with lemon) immediately after getting out of bed in the morning will stimulate a normal bowel movement.

4. Take a high fibre and roughage diet e.g. whole grain cereals and pulses, leafy vegetables like spinach, raw carrots, reddish, cucumber, salad, fruits like prunes, figs, papayas, oranges, water melon and other fresh fruits. Avoid refined and processed foods and foods with no fibre e.g. white flour ('Maida'), white sugar and their preparations, meats, egg, fish etc.

5. If constipation is very serious, take occasional 'enemas' but it shouldn't be made a regular habit because it will further discourage bowel movements. Enema should preferably be taken with lukewarm water and some mineral oil or glycerin can be mixed to it which will lubricate the walls of the colon. Enema should be taken with sufficient water so that water fills the colon properly and water should be retained for sufficient time so that hardened faeces soften down.

6. Daily physical exercise is beneficial for keeping the bowel movement in order. Bowel evacuation is stimulated by physical activity. It increases the **'peristalsis'** (wave like muscular movements taking place in the intestines for pushing forward the contents). This is why when a person gets up in the morning and does some physical activity, there develops a propulsive mass movement of the content of colon resulting in bowel evacuation.

7. Take green colour water. This water is prepared by keeping water in a green colour glass bottle in sunshine for about 8 hours. By this, water absorbs the green colour from sunrays. And this colour is good for removing constipation.

8. In case of severe constipation, purgatives or laxatives can also be taken but their regular use should be avoided because they promote inactivity of the intestines. Further herbal laxatives like 'Isabgol' are preferable to chemical laxatives. Mild laxative such as milk of magnesia should be preferred to strong laxative.

9. Do occasional fasting (by missing some meal off and on). During fasting body's entire energy becomes available for the purpose of elimination of waste, it (energy) being free from the task of digestion and hence you may find effective elimination of waste during such period. You can however drink plenty of water during such period to assist elimination, if possible by mixing a little lemon in it.

10. Gentle heat to the abdomen also increases peristalsis and aids in normal bowel movements.

11. Occasionally some oils like Olive oil, Castor oil or Almond oil may be used which will lubricate the walls of colon and also soften hard stool. But it shouldn't be used frequently as it absorbs and carries out of the body the fat soluble vitamins.

12. Indian method of squatting for latrine should be preferred than western style, because squatting applies natural pressure on your intestines and easily pushes the faecal matter forward. Those who use commode should have an 8" high stool to put feet on in order to bring the thighs up towards the abdomen so as to generate some pressure in lower abdomen.

13. Sit in Vajrasana (see Fig. 13.8) off and on and specially after eating food. Vajrasana increases the circulation in the abdomen and thereby increases the tone and efficiency of large intestines.

14. Consume eatables having lot of potassium e.g. banana, potato, tomato etc.

15. Drink water stored in Copper vessel while going to bed at night and at the time of getting up in the morning. Copper charged water is good in constipation.

Yoga Practices for Treatment of Constipation

(A) Shankh Prakshalan Kriya

In yoga there is a kriya called 'Shankh Prakshalan' which is very effective for clearing your bowels. In this kriya you first drink two glasses of warm water and then do the following exercises in sequence (each exercise to be done about four times for each side of the body). Then after doing all these exercises, again drink one glass of warm water and repeat the sequence of these exercises. Go on repeating the procedure till you get

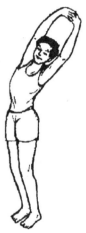

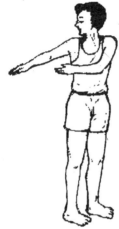

(A) Sideward bending by interlacing your fingers with stretched hands

(B) Rotation or lateral bending

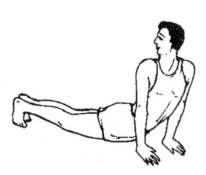

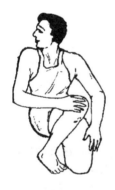

(C) Try to see your heels in this final position

(D) Touch the knee of one leg with the foot of another leg and also twist your body

Fig. 9.4

the motion. These exercises are designed in such a way that they contract, twist and bend the eliminative parts of our digestive system such that the waste or refuse is propelled forward.

(B) Miscellaneous Yogasanas for Relief in Constipation

Any kind of exercise or asana which alternately presses and releases your lower abdomen is good for constipation and the health of large intestine. 'Shankh Prakshalan' kriya mentioned earlier does this effectively but the following asanas can also ·be performed, preferably after drinking two glasses of water, for relief in constipation.

(i)   Pawanmuktasana   (ii)   Tadasana (or any other similar stretching of body)

(iii) Shashankasana   (iv) Makarasana

(v)   Uthanpadasana   (vi) Vajrasana

(vii) Paschimottasana

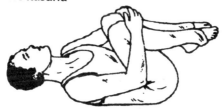

(i) Pawanmuktasana

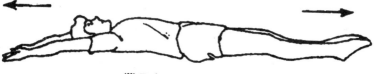

(ii) Tadasana (or any other similar stretching of body)

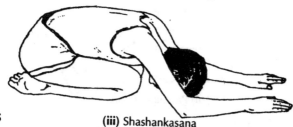

Fig. 9.5   (iii) Shashankasana

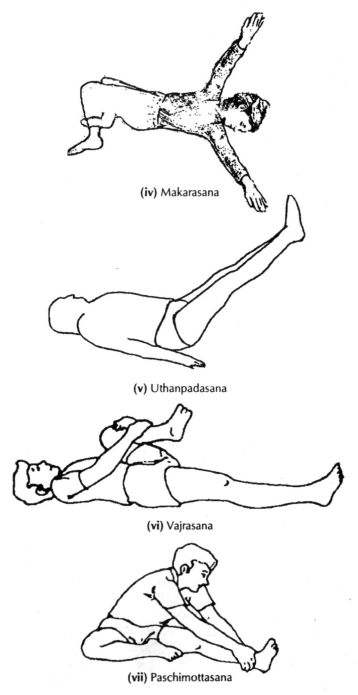

(iv) Makarasana

(v) Uthanpadasana

(vi) Vajrasana

(vii) Paschimottasana

Fig. 9.5 : Asanas for relief in constipation

In addition, Uddiyan Bandh and Mool Bandha are useful for relief in constipation. For details of these Bandhas see *Chapter 12* of the book.

(C) Pranayamas (Breathing exercises) for Constipation

Following Breathing exercises which focus on full and forced exhalation are good for relief of constipation e.g.

   (i) Kapalbhati Pranayama

   (ii) 'Gunjan' and 'OM' pranayam

   (iii) Nadi Shodhan pranayam

   (iv) 2 to 1 breathing (1 inhalation by nose, 2 exhalation by mouth)

   (v) Agnisara Pranayama

For details of these pranayamas see *Chapter 12* of the book.

(D) Abdominal Massage for Constipation

Lie down on your back, bend the knees, draw the legs and feet towards the buttocks. Now you have to massage or squeeze along your large intestine which is situated around your navel as shown in Fig. 9.6.

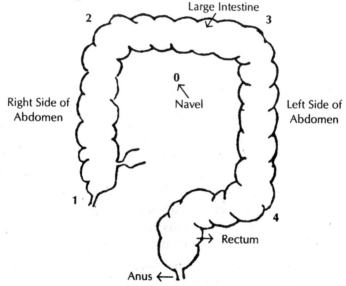

Fig. 9.6 : Abdominal massage along large intestine

See the nos. 1, 2, 3, 4 marked on this figure. Numbers 1 & 2 are the portions on the right side of the abdomen and 3 & 4 on the left side of abdomen. Now place your palm gently on point no. 1 and start massaging it by pressing and squeezing. Slowly move the palm towards position no. 2. Then proceed across the abdomen towards left side towards point no. 3. Now descend as you squeeze and massage and go to position no. 4 on the left side below the navel. Repeat the process five to six times starting once again from no. 1 position. This massage can also be easily practised while you are sitting on toilet bowl.

Some Home Remedies for Short Term Relief in Constipation

1. Take 'Isabgol' powder or 'Nature Care' (Dabur) with hot milk/hot water at night.
2. Take 'Trifala' or 'Harar' or 'Amla' powder with hot milk/hot water at night.
3. Take hot water mixed with salt just after getting up in the morning and walk briskly for few minutes before going for clearing bowels.
4. Take honey and lemon in hot water in the morning after getting up.
5. Take raisins ('Moonakka') after boiling in milk.
6. Take 'Gulkand' (M/s. Charak) with hot milk at night.
7. Take some ayurvedic formulations for bowel evacuation e.g. take 'Kabzahara' (M/s. Baidyanath) or 'Kabzola' (M/s. Tabex pharma Pvt. Ltd.) with water at night.
8. Take Castor oil in the night.
9. Cut a lemon into two halves. Apply some salt and black pepper on it and directly suck its juice in the mouth. Finish one full lemon.
10. Take 'enema' of lukewarm water in which some salt or lemon can be mixed. Readymade enema bags are also available nowadays in the market which can be easily used by the patient himself and later disposed of.
11. Take some allopathic laxative or purgative e.g. 'AGAROL', 'CREMAFFIN', DULCOLAX (tab).

10. Cancer

What is Cancer?

Cancer refers to any disorder of cell growth that brings about the invasion and destruction of surrounding healthy tissues by the abnormal cells. Cancer cells arise from normal cells whose nature has been permanently changed. They undergo multiplication more rapidly than healthy body cells and are not subject to normal control by nerves and hormones.

It may be noted that cancer is not one single disease but a term used to describe several diseases with the same general characteristics, and their causes and treatments are many and varied.

Nearly all the normal cell types may be transformed into a malignant or cancerous form.

S. No.	Type of Cells	After Becoming Malignant are Called as
1.	Epithelial cells	Carcinomas
2.	Connective tissue cells	Sarcomas
3.	Bone marrow cells	Leukaemia

How Cancer Spreads in the Body

Cancerous cells may spread via the bloodstream or lymphatic system to other parts of the body where they bring about further tissue damage (metastasis). Malignant tumours are a form of cancer. Leukaemia is cancer of white blood cells.

Warning Signals of Cancer

Watch out for the seven warning signals:

- Change in bowel or bladder habits
- A sore throat that does not heal
- Unusual bleeding or discharge
- Thickening or lump in breast or elsewhere
- Indigestion or difficulty in swallowing
- Obvious change in wart or mole
- Naggineg cough or hoarseness

Some Misconceptions and Their Clarifications about Cancer

1. Cancer is neither contagious nor communicable. It doesn't spread by germs. One can safely live and eat with cancer patient
2. Cancer can't be prevented or cured by any vaccination because vaccination works only for diseases caused by germs
3. Cancer is completely curable if detected at an early stage.

Detection of Cancer

For detection of cancer, initially the more general check ups are done such as:

i. Blood pressure and pulse

ii. Blood tests

iii. X-rays

iv. E.N.T. check up and other general physical/visual medical examination.

However some advanced medical tests used are:

i. Memography

ii. Zerography

iii. Thermography

iv. CAT Scan, MRI Scan

v. F.N.A.C. (Fine Needle Asperation Cytology)

vi. Biopsy

Causes of Cancer

The specific causes of cancer are still not fully understood. Scientists agree that most cancers are linked to how you live, what you eat, drink, breathe and smoke. Probable causative agents (carcinogens) are various chemicals, skin irritants, smoking and tobacco, silica and asbestos particles, free radicals, ionizing radiations (α-particles, γ rays, X-rays, ultraviolet rays), tarcoal etc. Hereditory factors and stress may also be important.

Prevention of Cancer

Here are some dietary and weight control tips that work as protective measures against the risk of cancer.

1. **Eat more Fresh Vegetables:** Studies show that certain kinds of vegetables (green and leafy or deep yellow) can help protect you against cancers of the colon, rectum, prostate, stomach, respiratory system, breast and cervix. Cabbage and cauliflower are especially beneficial.

2. **Add more High-Fibre Foods:** A diet rich in roughage is a safeguard against cancers of the colon and rectum. Some high-fibre foods are: brown bread, unpolished rice, whole wheat, cereal, popcorn, raisins, peaches, apples with skin, oranges, potatoes, spinach, peas and tomatoes.

3. **Choose Foods with Vitamin A:** These may help protect you against cancers of the oesophagus, larynx, mouth, stomach, colon, rectum, bladder and cervix. Vitamin A is found in egg yolk, dairy foods, fish, liver, fresh fruit (such as apricots, peaches and carrots) and green vegetables. It is far better to eat such foods than to take large quantities of vitamin tablets.

4. **Take more Vitamin C:** This may help ward off cancers of the oesophagus, mouth, colon, rectum, stomach and cervix. Some good sources are mangoes, cauliflowers, oranges, red and green chillies, tomatoes and strawberries.

5. **Take more Vitamin E:** Vit. A, C & E act as antioxidants and prevent cancer due to oxidative stress caused by free radicals. Some of the sources of Vit. E are — vegetable oils, green leafy vegetables, almonds, peanuts, walnuts,

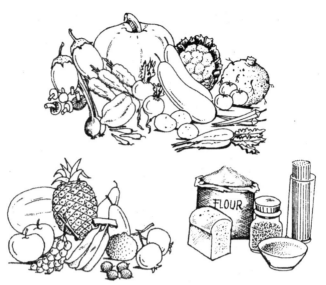

Fig. 11.1 Fresh fruits, vegetables and high fibre diet
are protective factors against cancer

egg yolk, whole grain cereals (specially wheat flour and wheat germ), milk, butter, onion, garlic, sprouted pulses.

6. **Miscellaneous Foods:** Some foods have been found specially good as cancer fighters such as — Lettuce, Tomatoes, Molasses, Turnips, Mushrooms, Cabbage, Figs, Selenium rich foods (onion, garlic, cucumber, radish etc.), Wheat grass juice, Grapes, Apricots, Almonds, Broccolisprouts, carrots, potatoes etc.

7. **Weight Control:** Obesity is linked to cancers of the colon, uterus, gall bladder and breast. Exercise and lower calorie intake help in keeping weight down. Walking is an ideal, enjoyable exercise. So are dancing, swimming, running and sports.

8. **Increase Immunity:** Increase the immunity and resistance power of your body by the measures given in Chapter 13.

Risks to Avoid in Daily Life

Scientists have noted that cancer is more prevalent among those used to certain practices and ways of life. Avoid these risk-enhancing factors, and you certainly improve your chances against the cancer threat.

1. **Trim Fat from Your Life:** A high-fat diet increases your risk of breast, colon and prostate cancer. Fat-loaded calories mean a weight gain for you, especially if you don't exercise. Cut over all fat intake by eating low-fat dairy foods, lean meat and fish. Eat chicken without the skin. Avoid high-sugar pastries and sweetmeats.

2. **Cut Down on Pickled, Barbecued or Salt Cured Foods:** Cancers of the oesophagus and stomach are common in countries where these foods are eaten in large quantities. Go easy on pickles and salt-cured fish and meats (such as bacon, ham and dried Bombay Duck).

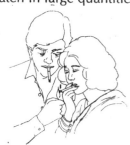

Fig. 11.2 Smoking can cause lung and bladder cancer

3. **Stop Smoking:** Smoking is the biggest cancer risk of all. It is the main cause of lung and bladder cancer. Smoking at home means more risk of cancer and respiratory ailments for those around you, including your family. Pregnant women who smoke harm their unborn babies.

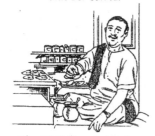

Fig. 11.3 'Paan' chewing can cause cancer of mouth and throat

4. **Stop Chewing Paan and Tobacco:** This is directly related to cancers of the mouth and throat, besides eroding teeth and gums.

5. **Go Easy on Alcohol:** If you drink a lot, your risk of liver cancer and cirrhosis increases. Smoking and drinking greatly increases risk of cancers of the mouth, throat, larynx and oesophagus. If you drink, be moderate.

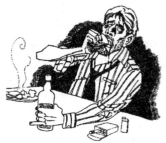

Fig. 11.4 Alcohol can cause liver cancer and cirrhosis

Cure of Cancer

Normally following treatments are resorted to for curing cancer:

i. Surgery

ii. Chemotherapy

iii. Radiation therapy (X-rays, γ rays, electrons, neutrons, protons etc.)

Surgery is helpful if the cancer is in the initial stages. Chemotherapy is a method of treating cancer or allied tumour growth with chemicals. Radiation therapy is the use of certain devices e.g. Cobalt Machine, Particle Accelerator and Linear Accelerator to treat cancer. With the help of all these treatments cancer cells are destroyed.

Stress and Cancer

With constant stress, **the adrenal glands** produce excessive amounts of **corticosteriods** that inhibit the normal surveillance operations of the immune system. The immunological actions of **macrophages**—the big oozing cells that repair damaged tissue, devour viruses, and engulf malignant cells—are impaired by these corticoid chemicals of stress. When people feel stressed, macrophage activity grows sluggish and immunity to disease falters. In addition the body's production of **'interferon'**, an anti-cancer substance originating in the cells, may also be impeded by excessive amounts of the adrenal stress hormones.

Further stress greatly affects the **'thymosins'**—beneficial secretions from the thymus gland which stimulate the maturation of immune cells. Thymus gland regularly produces those immunogenic T-cells that keep cancer and other diseases at bay. When its T-cells are not activated by the thymus hormone, abnormal cells may begin to proliferate and clinical cancer sets in. **Following a bout with severe stress, the thymus normally shrinks to half its size and millions of lymphocytes are destroyed.** Under continued chronic stress, so common in Western world life styles the thymus may remain in a shrunken, subfunctional condition and immunity to disease is lost.

11. AIDS

What is AIDS?

AIDS stands for 'Acquired Immuno Deficiency Syndrome'. It is a deadly disease for which no vaccine or specific treatment has yet been found despite the scale of research devoted to it throughout the world.

How is It Caused?

It is caused by a virus namely HIV (Human Immuno Deficiency Virus).

We are protected from diseases by our immune system. HIV virus destroys the immune system and the body becomes incapable of fighting off even the most benign infections. Hence HIV virus doesn't directly kill the person as such. It kills the person indirectly by creating other diseases due to loss of immunity.

HIV virus remains latent for many years after the person is infected. It can sometime take ten years for its symptoms to manifest.

Where Does HIV Live?

Our body is composed mostly of liquids. HIV lives in the blood, semen, vaginal fluid, menstrual flow and breast milk. When body fluids pass from one person to another, the virus can get passed on too.

How Does AIDS Spread?

The virus can spread in mainly three ways:

1. **Sex:** AIDS mainly spreads through sexual contact with an infected man or woman. It can also spread through infected semen in case of artificial insemination. Ideally sperm banks should screen the HIV status of donors.

2. **Blood:** Some medical procedures (injection, surgery) and other practices (tattooing, ear piercing, acupuncture, circumcision, etc.) can spread the virus if instruments coming into contact with the blood are infected with this virus. It can also be spread by blood transfusion if the blood so supplied is infected with this virus. Organ transplant may also spread this virus if organ of the donor is infected with HIV.

3. **Infected Pregnant Women:** A pregnant woman who is HIV infected can transmit the virus to her unborn child during pregnancy or during delivery. Infected mother can also transfer the virus to the infant via breast milk.

How to Identify an AIDS Patient

An AIDS patient is characterized by the following symptoms:

1. Loss of weight
2. Intermittent fever
3. Swollen glands
4. Night sweating and bodyache
5. White patches or ulceration in the mouth
6. Red spots and blisters on the skin.

Removal of some Misconceptions about AIDS

1. You can't tell by a person's appearance whether or not he or she is infected with HIV
2. You can be infected after a single act of intercourse
3. It doesn't spread through touch of AIDS infected person. It is perfectly safe to live, study, work and eat with a person who is HIV infected
4. AIDS virus can't live for more than 10 minutes outside the body. Hence it doesn't spread through any external objects or means.

Prevention of AIDS

Prevention is the only cure for AIDS.

1. Avoid all kinds of penetrative sex—vaginal, oral or anal with HIV infected person
2. Use condoms as a means of safer sex
3. Have sexual intercourse only with a faithful, uninfected partner (avoid multiple sex-partners)
4. Ensure that the syringe and needle are disposable or properly sterilized
5. Ensure that blood is tested before transfusion. Use blood that is certified 'HIV FREE'
6. Avoid pregnancy if infected with the HIV virus
7. Avoid commercial blood donations
8. Increase resistance power and immunity of body by the measures explained in Chapter 13

High-risk Groups for HIV Infection

The high-risk groups for HIV infection are:

1. Male homosexuals
2. Individuals indulging in anal intercourse
3. Commercial sex workers (CSW, prostitutes)
4. Promiscuous individuals with multiple sexual partners
5. Individuals who indulge in casual sex with strangers
6. I.V. (intravenous, mainliner's) drug abusers who share needles
7. People in the health care industry
8. Patients requiring repeated blood transfusion
9. Patients receiving inadequately screened blood from professional donors
10. Patients with sexually transmitted diseases (STDs)

Safe Sex and AIDS

Techniques that minimise the risk of contracting sexually transmitted diseases, including HIV infection, are termed safe practices. Sexual activity between two uninfected people is safe. Any sexual activity between two individuals (one or both of whom may be infected) which does not involve an exchange ot semen, vaginal fluids or any other contaminated body fluids is safe; e.g., use of condoms is considered a form of safe sex. One may safely indulge in non-oral, non-anal and non-coital sexual practices such as fondling, stimulation of erogenous zones, sensate focus exercises and penetration alternatives e.g., intercourse between the thighs, inter-mammary intercourse or mutual or self-masturbation. Masturbation is one of the best safe sex practices.

Some Questions Answered

Q. 1 Can kissing lead to HIV infection?

A. Dry kissing is considered safe. Wet kissing may be risky, as the virus is present in the saliva of infected persons. However, no confirmed cases of transmission through saliva have been reported so far (the presence of ulcers/ abrasions in the oral cavity increases the risk of contracting/transmitting the infection).

Q. 2 Isn't it likely that the virus can be transmitted by mosquito and insect bites?

A. No, the HIV virus cannot be transmitted by mosquito or insect bites.

Q. 3 Can HIV/AIDS spread through razors in a barber's shop?

A. Yes, it is possible. The razor can cause scratches and cuts on the skin that can lead to slight bleeding. If a blade that is HIV-contaminated is re-used on another individual, it can transmit the infection.

Q. 4 Can donating blood cause HIV infection in the donor?

A. Donating blood, as such, does not cause AIDS. However, blood donation should be done only at blood banks in recognised public hospitals, where sterile disposable equipment is used. Disposable needles should be used, which should be discarded after a single use, leaving no chance of transmitting the HIV infection.

Q. 5 Can homosexual contact cause AIDS?

A. Yes, if the other person is HIV infected.

Q. 6 Can anal or oral sex with a woman cause AIDS?

A. Yes, if the woman is HIV infected. Any exchange of body fluids is enough to cause HIV infection if the other person is HIV infected.

12. Increasing Resistance Power and Immunity of the Body

Your body has an inbuilt self healing mechanism. In a way it is its own Doctor. Because of this self healing property, even without your awareness most of the times body automatically takes care of various disease causing factors and doesn't allow you to become sick. However, this mechanism can become weaker or stronger depending upon how you maintain and look after your body. If you misuse your body, lead a faulty life style, self healing mechanism can soon break down and you can soon become prey to diseases very easily while other people may not fall ill under the same circumstances.

In this chapter we will investigate some of the ways by which you can quickly make up your lost vitality and increase your energy level which will automatically increase your power of resistance, self healing and immunity.

Although there are many ways to increase the body's stamina and power of resistance but we will describe here only some common methods which can be practised by a common man.

1. Pranayama (or Breathing Exercises)

According to Yogic science, our breath is directly related to 'Prana' or energy. The type of breath, its rhythm, its speed, its depth all these indicate the state of energy or Pranic flow in our body.

By doing various breathing exercises, we exercise our 'Prana' and make it strong. Breathing is the easiest tool with us to increase our energy level. Some of the breathing exercises are given below which one should do regularly to increase his vitality and energy level.

1. **Kapalbhati:** This pranayama consists of rapid and forceful exhalations which are carried out by contracting the abdominal muscles strongly and quickly. Make each exhalation as forceful as you can. Strive for short, explosive exhalation that can expel maximum air out of lung. Begin with 10–15 repetitions per round. Later increase the number of repetitions and number of rounds as your capacity increases. Don't increase the number of repetitions at the cost of vigour and speed of the exercise.

   Kapalbhati is a boon for increasing the fitness of cardiovascular system. An energetic practice (2 exhalations per second for one minute) accelerates the heart rate to a level that most people can achieve only by participating in vigourous sports. Kapalbhati, with minimum energy expenditure can give the same exercise and benefit to heart which are provided by Aerobic exercises. Kapalbhati results in robust circulation of blood and removal of large amount of volatile waste from the blood.

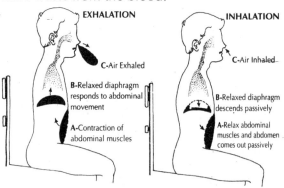

A-(Volume displaced by abdominal contraction) = **B** (Displacement of diaphragm) = **C** (Volume of air expelled)

A-(Volume recovered by relaxing abdominal muscles) = **B** (Displacement of diaphragm) = **C** (Volume of air inhaled)

Fig. 13.1 Kapalbhati Pranayama

2. **Nadi Shodhan Pranayama:** This pranayama is very helpful in balancing both components of your Autonomous Nervous System namely Sympathetic and Para Sympathetic Nervous system and thereby stabilize your mind.

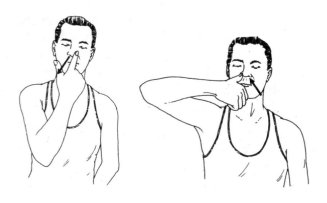

Fig. 13.2 Nadi Shodhan Pranayama

Shut your right nostril with the edge of your right thumb and inhale to a count of eight through the left nostril. Then close your left nostril with index finger and release your thumb from the right nostril and exhale to a count of eight from your right nostril keeping your index finger on the left nostril. Then begin inhaling again through the right nostril, reversing the sequence. This is one round. Do more rounds as per your capacity. Counts of inhalation and exhalation can be gradually increased as per your capacity but the ratio of inhalation and exhalation time should be maintained. This is a simplified form of Nadi Shodhan pranayama good enough for heart patients. Actual Nadi Shodhan pranayama as practised in yoga is a little different.

3. **'OM' Pranayama:** Inhale deeply and then exhale slowly through the mouth making the sound 'O'. Make this sound as loud and as lengthy as possible. Feel its vibrations spreading in the body. At the end close your lips making 'M' a humming sound.

4. **'Gunjan' Pranayama:** It is also called 'Brahmari Pranayamas'. Inhale deeply through both the nostrils and then exhale slowly through the nose only making sound of humming like a bee. Lips will remain closed.

5. **Bhastrika Pranayama:** It is same as Kapalbhati except that in Bhastrika both inhalation and exhalation are forceful. It is characterised by rapid and forceful inhalations and exhalations.

6. **2 to 1 Breathing:** This is very effective breathing exercise for increasing your vital power specially when you are tired. Here you inhale slowly from both nostrils and exhale slowly from mouth for twice the period of inhalation by keeping the lips partially open (as while whistling). You can practise this breathing anytime you feel exhausted or tired or while taking morning or evening walk in fresh air.

2. Aerobic Exercises

There is no parallel to aerobic exercises as far as increasing body stamina and power of resistance is concerned. Aerobic exercises involve rapid and continuous movements so that the rate of heart beats is increased and remains high for sometime. Exercises serving this purpose include brisk walking, running, cycling, swimming, jumping etc. The obvious benefit of these exercises is decrease in body weight by expenditure of excess calories and thereby reducing the work load of heart but the other important benefit is that these exercises strengthen the heart and lungs. Gradually after certain period of time you will find that your pulse rate has decreased for undertaking the same physical exertion. This means that your stamina has increased and the heart has become more efficient and is able to pump more volume of blood per beat (called stroke volume) and is

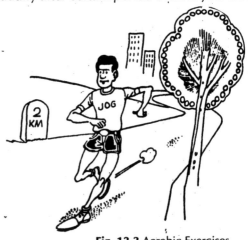

Fig. 13.3 Aerobic Exercises

therefore able to cope with the same physical strain with the smaller number of beats.

However, for getting proper benefit from Aerobic exercises, the pace of the exercises should be such that the pulse rate is raised to the target zone as indicated in the following table and remains in that zone for at least 15 minutes.

Table 13.1 Max. Pulse Rate during Physical Exercises

Age (in yrs)	Target Zone	Danger Zone
30–44	136–164	>170
35–39	132–160	>165
40–44	128–156	>160
45–49	124–152	>155
50–54	120–146	>150
55–59	116–140	>145
60–64	112–136	>140
65 and above	106–130	>135

Pulse rate shouldn't exceed beyond the danger zone during the exercises as mentioned in the above table. It should also be remembered that pulse rate should be raised gradually upto target zone by gradual warm up and similarly exercise shouldn't be stopped suddenly but should be gradually slackened and then stopped.

Persons with weak stamina will find that in the beginning they reach their target pulse rate by smaller physical exertion and exercise. Hence, initially they should limit themselves to such slow exercises such as brisk walking. Later as stamina · increases and pulse rate goes down for the same amount of physical exercise, they can increase their pace but again ensuring that their maximum pulse rate remains within the permissible zone and shouldn't cross danger zone.

As a thumb rule you can find your desirable maximum heart rate or pulse rate (for exercises) by subtracting your age from 180. The outward physical sign of achieving this heart rate is that you won't be able to carry out normal conversation at this heart rate (or pulse rate).

Exercises improve blood circulation and dilate the blood vessels and therefore help in efficient removal of waste products and toxins from the body.

3. Massage and Acupressure

Massage and acupressure are very effective means of balancing and strengthening the flow of energy (or Prana) in the body. In fact, when you are massaging you are also indirectly pressing some acupressure points. Similarly when you are giving acupressure at some points, you are also indirectly giving a deep pressure massage over the soft tissues (muscles etc.) of that area. By massaging the muscles, they get relaxed ensuring free circulation of blood and Prana. In acupressure, you press the points on acupuncture meridians because of which prana flow in meridians increases.

It is found that all the meridians end in the palms and soles of our body. According to principles of reflexology, all the parts of our body have reflex points in our palms and soles. Hence if you give acupressure and massage to your palms and soles of both sides, your whole body is energized. In fact, points in your soles and palms are like switches or buttons which when activated send the current or energy to those particular organs to which they correspond.

Hence for keeping your energy level high, you should once a day, give thorough massage or acupressure to the palms of your hands and soles of your feet. In winter it is all the more necessary. In winter you can do the same while sitting in sunshine and after applying some oil on hands and feet which will enhance the effect (see Fig. 13.4).

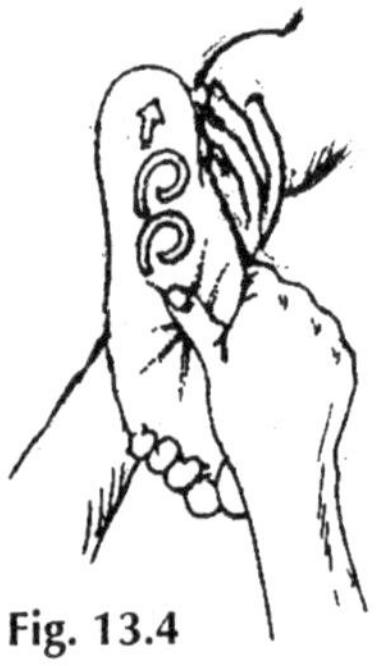

Fig. 13.4

You can give acupressure to the points in your foot and hand by specially available hand and foot roller now a days. (Fig. 13.5)

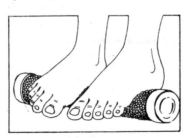

Fig. 13.5

176

There is one more important area for giving massage/acupressure for increasing the energy level of the body. It is on the back of body on both sides of spine. A very important acupuncture meridian (B1) runs on both sides of spine. It controls all other meridians. By giving acupressure on the points of these meridian your whole body is activated.

You can give the pressure on both sides of spine either in the form of continuous massage by your two fingers or thumbs after applying some oil or you can give pointed pressure by the thumbs of both hands as shown in the Fig. 6.31 in Chapter 6. You can also give acupressure on these points by using an acupressure roller as shown in Fig. 6.31A.

You can also give the massage to the whole of the back as shown below.

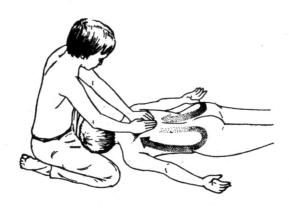

Fig. 13.6

4. Contact with Nature

Five elements of nature (air, water, earth, fire, sky) in their pure forms are a great source of energy for us. Whenever we are in physical contact with nature e.g. in the sun, enjoying natural bodies of water and lush vegetation or feeling the wind embracing us, we are absorbing this vital life force energy. Such deep nourishment from nature relaxes and rejuvenates. Fresh natural foods and trees also give us a lot of prana and rejuvenate us because they constantly absorb prana from these five

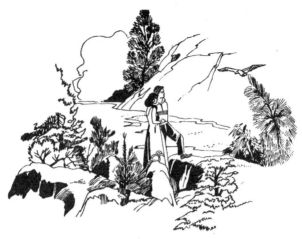

Fig. 13.7

elements of nature because of being in continuous contact with them. You might have observed how relaxing and rejuvenating it is to lie under the shade of big tree even in extreme summer.

Hence whenever you get time, go close to nature like gardens, forests, mountains, rivers, lakes etc. See the open sky, clouds and inhale fresh air. Listen to chirping of birds, play with children, listen to sound of moving breeze. Take healing ray of sun on your body.

5. Sitting Postures and Meditation

Meditation is the proven technique to increase one's energy level. Here it is your mind which is made use of for increasing the energy level of body as there is an intimate link between mind and body.

In meditation mind is made calm and still by focusing it on some neutral object so that it comes into what is called a state of 'Passive Awareness'. This focus can be anything like a visual object, a soothing sound, a mantra or your own breathing. The beginners usually find it convenient to focus their mind on their breath. While focusing on your breath, observe each inbreath and outbreath and notice how your abdomen swells during inhalation and how it falls during exhalation. This additional observation (falling and rising of abdomen) can assist one in being fully involved with the process. If mind deflects

178

from the focus, bring it gently to the focus again. While doing this meditation, the body should be completely comfortable, clothes should be loose, posture should be straight and balanced (preferably cross legged sitting postures or Vajrasana). If there is some discomfort in the body while sitting, it will not allow your mind to focus and calm down.

This perceptual process (of breath awareness or any other focus) immediately puts an end to any inner chatter going in your mind and makes it calm and still. When the mind becomes calm and still, energy or prana also becomes balanced because of its interrelationship with mind and whenever prana is balanced, it tends to be stronger.

Sitting postures especially designed for meditation are a further aid in calming your mind and balancing your energy or prana. This is because these postures enable spine to come in its natural straighter posture. The straight vertical spine encourages prana to be balanced and makes it rise upwards in 'Sushumna' nadi. Such flow of prana makes it quite strong and therefore your energy level rises.

Infact one easy way to instantly increase your energy level whenever you are feeling low is to just sit in 'Vajrasana' for a few minutes keeping your spine straight and eyes closed.

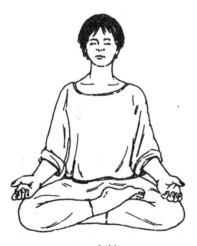 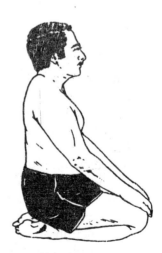

Sukhasana   Vajrasana

Fig. 13.8

179

6. Energy Locks

They are also called 'Bandhas' in the language of Yoga. They are special postures designed to conserve and make use of vast reserve of prana. They not only prevent dissipation of prana but also enable you to regulate its flow and convert it into spiritual energy. They are said to raise the latent Kundalini energy by their powerful effect on flow of prana. Practising these techniques will help you further in strengthening your energy level.

There are mainly three kinds of 'Bandhas' or 'Locks':

i. **Jalandhar Bandha:** While retaining your breath after inhaling, press your chin firmly into the chest. This prevents 'prana' escaping from upper body. Lift your head while you exhale.

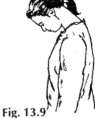

By pressing the chin against the chest, your 'Vishuddhi' chakra is activated with consequent stimulation of Prana.

Fig. 13.9
Jalandhar Bandha

ii. **Moola Bandha:** While retaining the breath, contract the anal sphincter muscles. This prevents the apana escaping from the lower body and helps in drawing it up to unite with prana. By 'Moola bandha' 'Mooladhara' chakra is activated which is a great generator of 'prana' in the body.

iii. **Uddiyana Bandha:** After exhaling completely, pull the abdomen back and up towards the spine as much as possible. By this 'Bandha', Solar Plexus or 'Manipura' chakra is activated which is a great reservoir of energy or prana in the body. You can also do 'Agrisara kriya' in this position. It consists of pumping the abdomen in and out while holding the breath in exhaled condition.

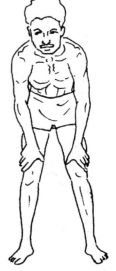

Fig. 13.10 Uddiyana Bandha

7. Prana Mudra

Bend the little and ring fingers so that their tips touch the tip (front edge) of thumb as shown in figure. It increases life force and cures nervousness and fatigue also helps increasing power of eyes. You can do this as many times as you like.

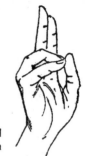

Fig. 13.11
Prana Mudra

8. Laughing, Dancing, Singing, Swaying, Clapping

Activities like laughing, dancing, singing, swaying in response to some good devotional music, rocking, swinging in a jhoola and clapping etc. done whole heartedly and spontaneously have a very positive effect on increasing your energy level as they lighten, open up and expand your mind. Hence try to include these things deliberately in your routine.

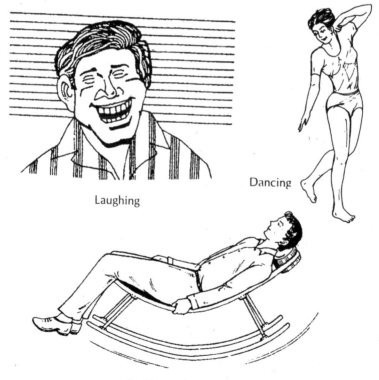

Laughing

Dancing

Rocking in a rocking chair

Fig. 13.12

181

9. Cold Water Bath

Cold water acts as a tonic for nervous system and increases the resistance power of the body. In summer, there is no problem in taking cold water bath. People invariably take it.

In winter when it is not possible to take continuous cold water bath, one can take hot water bath but it should always be concluded by cold water bath to get the desired benefit. Cold water increases the blood circulation, stimulates the sluggish nervous system and you will not feel shivering in winter after taking this bath.

13. Allergy

What is Allergy?

A llergy is abnormal hypersensitivity of the body cells to a specific substance which is normally harmless to an ordinary person. It results in various types of reactions in the body leading to various symptoms.

Types of Allergy

i. **Exogenic:** Caused by mainly external factors.

ii. **Endogenic:** caused by heredity or other internal factors.

Allergens

The substances that cause reaction in the body of allergic person are called allergens or antigens. While almost anything can be an allergen, some substances are frequent offenders as listed below–

i. Dust & pollution

ii. Pollens, plants

iii. Cosmetics & perfumes

iv. Certain foods like eggs, nuts etc.

v.   Preservatives ingested with food

vi. Industrial wastes, Automobile exhaust

vii. Sunlight

viii. Man-made fibres

ix. Certain drugs and vaccines

x.   Insecticides and pesticides

xi. Hair of certain animals, furs, mites etc.

xii. Paints (odour & smell).

Common Symptoms of Allergy

Most of the symptoms are elicited in the form of:

i. Inflammation/swelling accompanied or unaccompanied by pain

ii. Itching

iii. Redness and rise in temperature of the affected part

iv. Sneezing

v. Rashes on the skin

vi. Spotting on the skin.

Common Diseases Associated with Allergy

i. **Respiratory System:** Rhinitis, Sinusitis, Tonsillitis, Adenoiditis, Bronchial Asthma, Hay fever

ii. **Gastro Intestinal System:** Stomatitis, Peptic Ulcer, Flatulence, Diarrhoea, Abdominal cramps

iii. **Musculo-skeletal System:** Arthritis, Myalgia, Spondylosis

iv. **Skin:** Eczema, Dandruff, Urticaria, Acne (pimples), Psoriasis, Alopecia, Pruritus Vulvae, Dermatitis

Some Useful Notes about Allergy

1. Allergy is a reaction of the body to a harmless substance. Substance like pollens of the flowers, spores of fungi, house dust, eggs, fish, wheat or nickel, chromium and penicillin are harmless to all people, except those who are allergic to them. Pollens, fungal spores and house dust can cause recurrent bouts of sneezing or asthma; foods like eggs, fish, wheat can cause rashes, cramps in the abdomen and diarrhoea; nickel and chromium can cause reaction in the skin (contact dermatitis) and penicillin can cause anaphylactic reaction in which there is sudden collapse of the person allergic to it.

2. The substance that causes reaction in an allergic person is called allergen or antigen. The substance produced in the body of an allergic person as a result of the introduction of an allergen or antigen is called antibody. When antigen

and antibody meet together and react, the process is called antigen—antibody reaction.

3. In allergic reactions (antigen-antibody reaction) substances like histamine, serotonin and many others are released. These are the substances which cause the manifestation of allergy, like spasm of the muscles of the lung airways in asthma, or exudation of fluid from the nasal mucous membrane in cases of seasonal sneezing or irritation, swelling and redness of the skin in cases of urticaria etc.

4. Drugs in the group of 'Antihistamines' work by acting against and destroying histamine that is produced in allergic reactions. 'Avil', 'Phenergan', 'Actifed', 'Zyncet', 'Recofast', 'Cetrizen' are some examples of 'Antihistamines' or anti-allergic drugs.

5. The anaphylaxis allergic reaction is a particular type of severe allergic reaction, which can be life-threatening since the lungs may be so badly affected that asphyxiation occurs; immediate medical attention is essential. Anaphylatic shock can occur as a response to certain drugs, such as aspirin, penicillin and some foods also, but fortunately it is rare.

6. Allergy is inherited also but what is inherited is allergy and not a particular manifestation of allergy. For example, a parent may have asthma and his one son may have eczema and another a tendency to get sneezing. Similarly a person may have eczema in childhood, develop sneezing when he grows up and then may have asthma instead of these manifestations or over and above them.

Treatment of Allergy: There is as such no permanent cure for allergy. The best way to get rid of allergic reactions is to find out what one is allergic to and then to avoid contact with it. However, if one increases his resistance power and immunity of his body by measures given in Chapter 13, he can face this problem with much ease and less suffering.

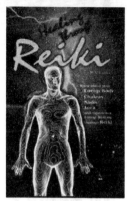

Healing Through Reiki
—M.K. Gupta

Contrary to what some people believe, Reiki is not a shady practice rooted in unfounded principles, but a systematic healing therapy based on the universal life force that pervades the entire cosmos. The Japanese refer to this invisible but universal energy as *Ki*, the Chinese as *Chi*, while Indians term it *prana*.

This energy forms an invisible pranic form around our physical body. This pranic form provides energy to the physical body and any disturbance in the pranic form affects our physical body, causing various ailments. Reiki is the science of tapping this pranic energy and using it to heal and nourish the physical body. Correcting any energy imbalance in the pranic form automatically heals the corresponding physical body.

In this book, the author highlights the association between the Japanese-discovered Reiki and the Indian healing techniques based on *chakras, nadis* and Yoga. The book also outlines Reiki attunement or the process of empowerment. With many photos and illustrations, the book reveals Reiki treatment for specific ailments.

Demy Size • Pages: 104
Price: Rs. 60/- • Postage: Rs. 15/-

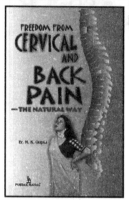

Freedom from Cervical and Back Pain
—M.K. Gupta

Two of the most incapacitating ailments in modern times are cervical pain and backache. Both ailments can severely hamper a person's movement, denting the patient's personal and professional life. There is no permanent cure in allopathy for both ailments. Painkillers and other medications simply provide temporary relief... until the next spasm of excruciating pain shoots through the body again.

The book puts all relevant issues regarding the two ailments in proper perspective. At the outset, it highlights the proper postures that can help prevent backache and cervical pain. It also lists the precautions to be taken while exercising.

Patients are then taught how to find relief through the practice of Yoga. If practised regularly with patience and diligence, Yoga can provide permanent relief to patients. The book tells readers how to maintain good posture and perform loosening and strengthening exercises for the muscles that gradually restore the tone and alignment of these muscles before degenerative and irreversible damage occurs.

Demy Size • Pages: 128
Price: Rs. 68/- • Postage: Rs. 15/-

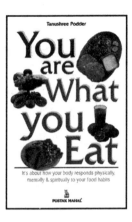

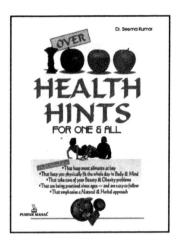

You are
What you Eat
—Tanushree Podder

It's about how your body responds
physically, mentally & spiritually to
your food habits

Did you know that food could heal,
cure, elevate moods, improve memory,
make the brain sharper, provide us with
potent energy and fill us with vigour?

Food has been discovered to be the greatest
natural pharmacy that is available to
human beings. The right food can help us
perform to our peak capacity while the
wrong food can lead us towards disease
and ill health.

The ordinary cabbage and cauliflower
could ward off the possibility of cancer,
tomatoes can effectively take care of free
radicals in today's environment and carrots
can provide you with the essential beta-
carotene to fight off many diseases. It is
surprising how effectively food can alleviate
most of our common ailments.

The mysteries of the power of food and
the secrets of food elements have been
unravelled so that you can use food for
other benefits rather than just appeasing
hunger.

Demy Size • Pages: 184
Price: Rs. 80/- • Postage: Rs. 15/-

Over 1000 **Health Hints**
for one & all

—Dr. Seema Kumar

With ever-rising ground, water and
atmospheric pollution, every other day,
one hears the name of a new disease.
Today, we breathe air thick with exhaust
fumes, eat processed junk food that has
no nutritive value, drink toxic carbonated
beverages and lead sedentary lives. All of
this ensures that we are plagued with
different kinds of problems at regular
intervals.

This book shows you how to go back to
Mother Nature to beat even the most
troublesome and chronic ailments. With
natural preventive measures that
emphasise diet, exercise and herbal
remedies, there are no fears of obnoxious
side effects.

Whatever be your problem—diabetes,
blood pressure, asthma, acne, menopause,
obesity, stomach ailments, premature
ageing or general complaints—this book
shows you a safe, natural and enjoyable
means to overcome it. Most of the
ingredients mentioned in the book are
the kind available in home gardens or off
the kitchen shelf.

Big Size • Pages: 168
Price: Rs. 80/- • Postage: Rs. 15/-

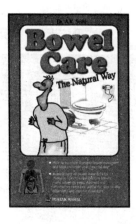

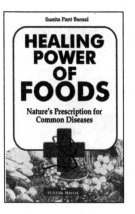

Bowel Care
The Natural Way

—Dr. A.K. Sethi

Good digestion is the key to a healthy body and sound mind. Considering today's eating habits, modern lifestyle and the stress and tension of hectic schedules, most of us suffer from digestive problems. In many cases, however, a person needs the right information and a little care in regulating his/her dietary habits and lifestyle.

Bowel Care is especially designed as an ideal self-help guide to all who suffer from such problems—or are likely to. Presented in an easy, lucid style with lively illustrations, it brings home to the reader a "Total Solution".

Written by a specialist in his field, it is a well-researched and simple work to provide relief to the readers.

The book highlights:

❖ Structure and functions of the Digestive System and related organs ❖ Causes and symptoms of bowel disorders ❖ Diagnosis and treatments of common digestive ailments ❖ Management of bowel disorder through Diet, Yoga, Meditation and Ayurvedic treatments.

Demy Size • Pages: 112
Price: Rs. 60/- • Postage: Rs. 15/-

Healing Power of FOODS

—Sunita Pant Bansal

Hippocrates, the father of medicine, recognised that the medical therapy must be consistent with the nature and the design of the human body. He believed that the effective health care could not be separated from nutrition. He stressed prevention of disease by strongly recommending a balanced diet with a moderate and sensible lifestyle. Hippocrates wrote, "Natural forces within us are the true healers of disease... Everything in excess is opposed to nature... To do nothing is sometimes a good remedy." His philosophy was very much akin to the holistic health perspective of today.

The various foods provide not only nutrition to our body, but can prove to be medicinal too. *Healing power of Foods* introduces all the main food groups to the reader, giving details about the medicinal uses of the commonly used foods from these groups. The tips given are simple, practical and effective. The healthy recipes at the end of the book complete the role of the various foods in providing nutritional as well as medicinal benefits.

Demy Size • Pages: 136
Price: Rs. 80/- • Postage: Rs. 15/-

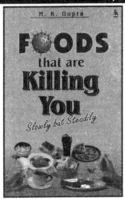

FOODS
that are Killing You
—M. K. Gupta

It is truly said: *You are what you eat.* Although most of us have heard this axiom, we don't bother to give it a second thought. That is why, white sugar, table salt, fatty and acidic foods and the wrong food combinations, besides other pesticide-laden foods, are part of our everyday menu.

Foods that Are Killing You seeks to increase awareness among readers about wrong eating habits that end up destroying our health and silently killing us. The book also highlights the dangers of consuming coffee, tea, alcohol and milk – yes, milk!

The harmful effects of all these foods are explained in explicit terms. Proper scientific understanding of the side effects of such harmful foods can ensure that we eliminate or control the consumption of foodstuffs containing excess pesticides and cholesterol, leading to enhanced well-being and better health. This book is a must in every home, because health is truly wealth.

Demy Size • Pages: 160
Price: Rs. 80/- • Postage: Rs. 15/-.

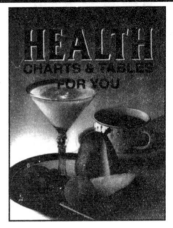

HEALTH CHARTS
& Tables for You
—M.K. Gupta

As any health-conscious person knows, health is truly wealth. Yet, simply harbouring good intentions does not ensure good health for anyone. Beginning in infancy and right up to our twilight years, a conscious attempt has to be made to lead a healthy lifestyle. In the formative years, our parents make this effort on our behalf. But as we enter the teens and take control of our own destinies, how well informed we are on health-related issues makes all the difference between physical well-being and ill health.

This book ensures you have all the facts, figures and data at your fingertips to promote proper health and nutrition in order to prevent disease.

In this book you will find: height and weight charts, blood pressure and pulse rate charts, calorie charts, fat and cholesterol charts, vitamin and mineral charts, balanced diet charts, pollution health hazard charts, infectious diseases and immunisation charts, healthy heart and stress charts... not to mention other relevant charts, tables and data.

Big Size • Pages: 144
Price: Rs. 96/- • Postage: Rs. 15/-

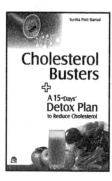

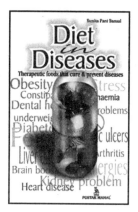

Cholesterol Busters

A 15-Days' Detox Plan to Reduce Cholesterol

—Sunita Pant Bansal

Over the past decades there has been a growing concern world over about the higher deposits of cholesterol in human body resulting in life-threatening diseases in millions of people. The solution is to understand the genesis of the problem and devise ways to be free from it.

The author opines that it is not only higher intake of fats but other factors such as excess weight, lack of exercise, alcohol, smoking and stress which lead to high level of cholesterol in human body. She further focuses on cholesterol-busting food and suggests a fifteen-days DETOX programme yielding fantastic results in 6-8 weeks.

Pages: 104
Price: Rs. 60/- • Postage: 15/-

Diet in Diseases

—Sunita Pant Bansal

Diet plays a crucial role in promoting or preventing a disease. Especially when down with a disease, simply swallowing pills will not prove as effective if dietary guidelines are ignored. The appropriate therapeutic diet can speed up the recovery process and even boost the immune response. However, diet is one aspect of therapy that even doctors many a times fail to give due importance to. Simply put, over-nutrition, under-nutrition or wrong nutrition must equally be avoided if one wishes to stay slim, trim and fighting fit.

This book lists an array of ailments and conditions and outlines the right diet that could cure or control these problems. Once you begin having balanced, sensible meals, it won't be long before you kiss goodbye to those pills. This book will show you how to eat right and stay fit.

Demy Size • Pages: 104
Price: Rs. 69/- • Postage: Rs. 15/-